Parkinson Positive

STRENGTH FOR THE JOURNEY

Jerry Gill and Bruce McIntyre

D1294546

Prairie Wind Press

Stillwater, Oklahoma

Parkinson Positive

Copyright © 2015 by Prairie Wind Press LLC

ISBN 978-0-692-55028-1

Printed in the USA by Prairie Wind Press, LLC

Contents

Dedication

This book is dedicated to Susan Gill, caregiver, life-long partner, and loving mother and grandmother,

Also to Kathy McIntyre who encourages and inspires many people while living with chronic illness,

And to the individuals with Parkinson's and their caregivers who have touched our lives and inspired us to share their message of hope.

Acknowledgments

Many individuals have accompanied us on our *Parkinson Positive* journey. We acknowledge their encouragement and contributions.

First of all, Rachel Cunningham edited out the many spelling and grammatical errors that crept into the manuscript and provided helpful editorial suggestions. Brandon Sayre transformed our vague concepts of layout and design into an inviting and readable format. And we thank Tim Watson for capturing the tone and spirit of this book with an excellent cover design.

We also recognize the special contribution of Monte Akridge, who has inspired us with his strong Christian faith and is a role model for the power and importance of faith in living successfully with Parkinson's.

Dr. Dean Shipley, Jim Keating, Christina Santos, Glenn Norris, and Tanya Bryant gave us helpful feedback on the initial manuscript. We are grateful for their insightful suggestions for improvement.

To Jim Keating, founder of the Parkinson Foundation of Oklahoma, and to the Foundation, we acknowledge their support and encouragement that helped make this book possible.

Finally, we extend our love and appreciation to our families and many friends who encouraged us throughout our journey.

Introduction

Hope and informed optimism are overarching themes of this book. Being diagnosed with Parkinson's disease is no happy event, but neither is it cause for despair. You have deep emotional and spiritual reserves that can help lift you and sustain you on your journey with Parkinson's. The authors affirm Helen Keller's words and resolute spirit: "The world is full of suffering. It is also full of overcoming it."

Parkinson Positive is a primer, a "101 course," on Parkinson's written for lay people. It provides basic information on causes and symptoms of this disease and current medical and therapy treatments. And as the title suggests, it is an informative guide to living successfully and positively with Parkinson's.

It is not intended to be a scholarly or comprehensive treatise on all aspects of Parkinson's, though it contains much valuable information. For in-depth information, we encourage you to consult sources cited in the text and "Endnotes" and the "Recommended Resources" listed in the appendix.

The authors' perspectives derive from their real life experiences and daily interaction with Parkinson's patients and their families. Bruce is the Executive Director of the Parkinson Foundation of Oklahoma. Jerry has lived with Parkinson's since being diagnosed in 2010 and serves on the board of directors of the foundation.

We have presented programs and participated in support groups and conferences across Oklahoma. And in turn, we have been blessed by our interaction and conversations with hundreds of people with Parkinson's and their caregivers. We have heard their stories, shared their pain, and been inspired by their courage and resilience.

Our work also has brought us into contact and relationship with compassionate, highly skilled doctors and health care professionals who specialize in the treatment of Parkinson's patients. This book is informed by our relationships with these patients and professionals.

Our collective experiences and personal conversations have revealed that there remains much misinformation and misunderstanding about Parkinson's, resulting in needless despair. We will shine a light into the darkness of uncertainty and unknowing to expose myths and to help you live *Parkinson Positive*.

This book is co-authored within the shared context and experiences of both authors. However, the text of the chapters varies according to the writing style of each author. The introduction and conclusion as well as chapters one, five, and seven are written by Jerry. Bruce is the author of chapters two, three, four, and six. All chapters include input from both authors.

Vignettes inserted at the beginning of each chapter are not true stories, but they contain universal truths about the emotional impact of Parkinson's commonly shared by patients and their caregivers. Hopefully, they will help you understand that your questions, doubts, and fears (real and perceived) are not unique to you.

Information on medications and other medical interventions mentioned in this book are included to help educate. They are not intended to offer professional advice or make claims about the appropriateness or effectiveness of any medication or medical procedure.

You should consult your doctor and other health care team members before making any decisions about managing or modifying your medical protocols. The authors do not endorse or make any warranties regarding health care and other information cited in this book.

In *Parkinson Positive* you will gain valuable knowledge about Parkinson's disease. This information will empower you to proactively participate in decisions concerning your medical treatments. The importance of a self-managed approach to Parkinson's disease is stressed throughout the book. This patient-centric model offers opportunity and imposes responsibility for you to manage your disease.

Parkinson's patients who are better informed about their disease have better outcomes. Knowledge is powerful medicine when prescribed with hope. In *Parkinson Positive* you will discover strength and courage to sustain that hope on your life long journey with Parkinson's. We invite you to join us on that journey of self-discovery.

CHAPTER 1

Devastating News

I have no choice about whether or not I have Parkinson's; I have nothing but choices about how I react to it.

—MICHAEL J. FOX

J ohn's worsening symptoms had finally precipitated a doctor's appointment. In anticipation of that doctor's visit, John busied himself with projects and diversions. Mary poured her energy into research. But the fear of the unknown lay beneath the surface of every smile, every meal, and every daily habit.

Finally, the day of the appointment arrived. After the doctor delivered the news, he stepped out of the room for a moment.

"Did the doctor say that he thinks I have Parkinson's?" John asked with a whisper.

"I'm afraid so, honey," Mary replied with a look of disbelief.

They drove home in silence, absorbing what this news might mean. From worst-case scenarios to unrealistic hopes of a misdiagnosis, their minds raced along similar tracks.

Devastating News

My (Jerry's) response to being diagnosed with Parkinson's was perhaps similar to yours. Initially, I experienced some unexplained troubling symptoms: slight tremors in one hand, smaller and less legible handwriting, difficulty remembering, and voice quality deterioration. "Really nothing to worry about," I told myself. "It's just aging or some temporary condition that will go away."

After having ignored these symptoms for several months, I took the advice of my primary care physician to seek further medical consultation. Next, I met with my orthopedic doctor, thinking that my tremors and handwriting were related to rotator cuff and sciatic nerve problems for which I had previously been treated. He examined me and assured me that nerve damage was not the source of my problem. Then we discussed my symptoms. Afterwards, he consulted with my primary care doctor, and they referred me to a neurologist with experience treating Parkinson's patients. "Parkinson's disease," I murmured to myself. My anxiety level increased exponentially.

After examining and observing me over a period of nearly a year, my neurologist confirmed my worst fears. "You have Parkinson's disease." I was devastated. Emotions of disbelief, denial, and fear flooded my mind, followed by a torrent of questions. What is Parkinson's disease? Why did this happen to me? How did I get this disease? How many years of quality life, if any, can I expect? Should I start now on my "bucket list" of things to do before I die? What do I say to my family, friends, and colleagues?

And perhaps my greatest fear and ultimate disappointment was how this was going to change my life and how others perceived me. I had participated in multiple sports in high school and received a football scholarship at a major university. During my professional career, I had regularly worked sixty to eighty hours a week. My self-esteem was in many ways tied to these accomplishments. Would I now be an invalid subject to falling down, confined to a wheel chair, and dependent on others?

Likely, you experienced similar emotions. Perhaps, earlier in your life, you had been a dancer, gymnast, active independent person, tireless worker, caregiver for your family, successful business person or professional, and a person others looked to for strength and support. Now, seemingly robbed of your dignity and self-worth, how will you respond?

Early Diagnosis and Intervention

We are not alone. It is estimated that up to 1.5 million Americans are living with Parkinson's disease. Approximately 50,000 to 60,000 new cases are diagnosed annually, and the total number of cases worldwide is expected to double to 30 million by 2030. Parkinson's is the second most common neurological disease. Most Parkinson's patients are diagnosed in their 60s, but approximately 15% are diagnosed before the age of 40. Parkinson's for this younger population is commonly referred to as "early onset" Parkinson's.

It is tempting and certainly understandable to bemoan your condition, and ask, "Why me? Why am I one of the 'unlucky' 2% to 4% of the general population that has Parkinson's?" The reality is that at this time there is no definite answer. You can have a pity party, but the problem with pity parties is that nobody wants to attend. Perhaps a more appropriate question is, "Why not me?" Bad things happen to good people, and none of us are exempt. Having Parkinson's is chance; how you live with it is choice. You have Parkinson's, but it doesn't have you. You are not defined by your disease. You are defined by the way you live your life—with courage, dignity, hope, and love.

Early diagnosis and treatment of Parkinson's are critical. While I didn't realize it at the time, I was fortunate to have two compassionate and knowledgeable doctors. They listened to me, considered my symptoms, collaborated, and referred me early in my disease to a neurologist who worked with Parkinson's patients.

Many Parkinson's symptoms are similar to and sometimes confused with other diseases and medical conditions. The collective commonality of these disease symptoms is often referred to as "parkinsonisms." In addition to Parkinson's, these symptoms are observable, in varying degrees, in essential tremor, dementia, strokes or brain tumors, amyotrophic lateral sclerosis (ALS), commonly referred to as Lou Gehrig's disease, and multiple system atrophy (MSA). Early diagnosis is critical. Unfortunately, it can be two or more years before patients are referred to a neurologist specializing in movement disorders and properly diagnosed. This is precious time lost in treating this progressive disease.

Consultation with doctors and health care professionals who have experience working with Parkinson's patients can help you better understand the trajectory of the disease and develop strategies for early intervention. Your first step should be to find a neurologist with whom you feel comfortable and confident. Next to yourself, this physician will be the most important member of your health care team. He or she will be critical in helping you jump-start your medical protocols, as well as develop and monitor your ongoing medical treatment plan.

There are several sources that can help you find a neurologist who specializes in movement disorders and has experience working with Parkinson's patients. And if you are not comfortable with the first physician you select, choose another one. It is important that you have confidence in and can develop a good working relationship with your neurologist. You will find information in chapter two and in the "Selecting A Physician" worksheet in the appendix to assist you in finding a physician that is right for you.

There are other key actions you will want to consider early in your intervention strategy. Jim Keating, founding director of the Parkinson Foundation of Oklahoma (PFO), emphasizes that the period immediately following the diagnosis is crucial to development and early implementation of your treatment plan.

"Generally, the neurologist will discuss symptoms with the patient, prescribe medications, and set up appointments spaced a few months apart. An important early role of PFO for supporting newly diagnosed patients is to fill these gaps between doctor visits. PFO can provide patients with educational information and services that help them and their families better understand the disease and consider additional strategies to complement their medication plan. For example, the PFO offers an introductory 'Parkinson 101' class and individual family consultations. These sessions provide basic information, direct participants to additional resources, and refer them, as needed, to other health care services."

Keating notes, "The Parkinson Foundation of Oklahoma also hosts educational conferences featuring nationally prominent speakers and provides resource people for support group meetings across the State. And we partner with health care organizations to offer voice therapy and Parkinson's specific exercise programs."

We encourage you to connect with a Parkinson organization near you. Many state, regional, and national organizations offer similar services.

Knowledge is Powerful Medicine

For many, the most devastating emotional impact of Parkinson's is the unknown. Every individual experiences the disease differently—different disabilities, different degrees of severity, and different rates of progression. Currently, there is no known prevention or cure. But many people with Parkinson's, through early intervention, including proper medication, therapy, and healthy lifestyle, can mitigate the severity of symptoms and enjoy a quality life, often for many years.

There is much misinformation and misunderstanding about Parkinson's in the public arena. Let's start with a common one. The first question often asked by newly diagnosed Parkinson's patients is, "How long can I expect to live?" Surprisingly, research studies indicate that the life expectancy of people with Parkinson's is only slightly less (approximately two to three years) than people without Parkinson's. The authors of *Navigating Life with Parkinson Disease* contend, "It is not unusual for many people who have lived with Parkinson's disease for many years to die 'with' rather than 'from' Parkinson's."

The question, correctly posed, is then not how many years of life do I have remaining, but rather, how much life do I have in my remaining years? Your challenge is to implement medical and lifestyle strategies that will help you sustain quality of life throughout your life.

Your Parkinson's diagnosis is not a death sentence.

Research on the symptoms and treatment of Parkinson's is offering patients hope for both long and productive lives.

The next step is to become better informed about your disease. This will include current medicines, therapies, and medical procedures to treat the symptoms of Parkinson's.

You are the most important member of your team.

You need to become knowledgeable enough to communicate clearly and effectively with your physician and other health care providers. Knowledge is powerful medicine.

There are many excellent resources to help you better understand the disease and implement a personal plan for living positively with Parkinson's. State and national Parkinson's foundations and organizations maintain websites that include blogs, articles on current research, and other valuable information. Many of these organizations also host conferences, workshops, and support groups that offer valuable suggestions for living with Parkinson's. Professional societies, like the American Academy of Neurology, provide information on current research. Research studies funded by hospitals, universities, and government agencies also should be consulted.

Doctors and other health care professionals who work with Parkinson's patients are excellent sources of information and can refer you to helpful resources. Don't overlook members of support groups and individuals living successfully with Parkinson's. They have years of experience and practical advice that they can share with you. Individuals and companies that provide services and products to persons with Parkinson's also can be helpful sources for information. Books and other publications, in print or electronic format, are additional sources to consult. Many of the sources cited above are referenced in the "Endnotes" and "Recommended Resources".

What Is Parkinson's and What Causes It?

As indicated earlier,

> *Parkinson's is a complex disease that affects each patient differently*

and with different outcomes. The array of possible disorders and disabilities of the disease can be physically and emotionally overwhelming. Much remains unknown about the disease and what causes it. Why do some people develop Parkinson's and others not? Why do they experience different disabilities and different degrees of severity? While there are currently few definitive answers, research is providing information that is helping us understand and more effectively treat Parkinson's.

Two primary factors are related to the onset of Parkinson's—a genetic predisposition and an activating event. Judith Stern, researcher at the University of California, explains that,

> *"...genes load the gun, and the environment pulls the trigger."*

Exactly which genes cause an individual to be susceptible to Parkinson's and what environmental factors trigger the onset of the disease are currently unknown. But current research in these areas is providing answers and offering hope for interventions that someday will prevent onset or stop the progression of this disease.

Information in this book will address questions and provide basic information about Parkinson's in language that lay people can comprehend. For individuals desiring in-depth information, we suggest that you refer to the "Recommended Resources".

Simply stated,

> *Parkinson's disease is caused by deficiency of "dopamine" in the brain.*

This deficiency occurs primarily in the region referred to as the substantia nigra located at the top of the brain stem. People are born with a defined set of brain cells, or neurons, and unlike other cells in the human body, neurons cannot regenerate themselves. Through the normal process of aging brain cells die, but a sufficient number of neurons remain to ensure functionality. However, in Parkinson's, neurons die sooner and more frequently. For example, this estimate is telling.

From 60% up to 80% of neurons have been lost before the first symptoms are observable in Parkinson's patients.

Neurons communicate with each other through electrical signals transmitted from one cell to another by a chemical they secrete called a neurotransmitter. The complex process of transmitting just one message may engage hundreds or even thousands of neurons. However, neurons will communicate only through neurotransmitters specific to their circuit or functional group of cells. Dopamine is an important neurotransmitter produced by neurons in the substantia nigra of the brain.

A major role of dopamine in the substantia nigra is to communicate to an area of the brain called the striatum. Programming for movement (walking, for example) occurs in the striatum. And in turn, the stratium communicates messages to motor centers of the brain that control muscles related to movement. When cells in the substantia nigra degenerate, dopamine secreted by these cells declines precipitously and is insufficient to effectively transmit information to the striatum and subsequently to other motor centers. At this point the communication cycle breaks down. This domino effect results in the inability of the motor centers of the brain to properly control motion and movement.

Dopamine deficiency in the substantia nigra-striatum (nigrostriatal) system affects movement, but other brain circuits are also impacted by loss of dopamine. The autonomic nervous system operates automatically without a person's conscious thought. It regulates the function of many internal organs including: heart, lungs, liver, stomach, intestines, bladder, reproductive organs, and salivary glands. Symptoms caused by loss of dopamine in this system are not as observable as motor symptoms, but they can create serious health issues. Some of these will be discussed later.

What causes neurons to die is not completely understood, but research has provided some tantalizing clues. A factor common to the degeneration of neurons is the presence of clusters of damaged proteins, commonly referred to as Lewy bodies. These are named for Dr. Frederick Lewy, who first observed them in 1913. Recent research indicates that a brain protein, alpha-synuclein, is highly concentrated in Lewy bodies and suggests a strong causal relationship. Still unanswered are why this abnormality occurs, why some individuals are genetically predisposed to this degenerative process, and what triggers it.

Parkinson's Disabilities

Parkinson's is a frustratingly complex disease. It creates a wide array of physically, mentally, and emotionally debilitating disorders that at best challenge quality of life and at worst are life threatening.

Parkinson's is progressive, and currently there is no known prevention or cure.

However, for many individuals, the severity of symptoms can be lessened and managed. But we come late to the battle. Early intervention is critical, but as indicated earlier, it's not until approximately 60% to 80% of our dopamine is lost that we even know we have Parkinson's. It's like playing a football game without a scoreboard and not knowing until the fourth quarter that you are behind, way behind.

The litany of Parkinson's symptoms is formidable and lengthy.

They include movement and motor disorders, cognitive and mental disabilities, speech and voice quality problems, and other related non-motor symptoms. Functions associated with normal aging are exacerbated by Parkinson's. Cognitive functions weaken and slow down, ordinary tasks take longer to complete, multi-tasking is more difficult, and social and interpersonal skills are reduced.

Movement and motor functions are the most common and observable disabilities of Parkinson's. Tremors (initially on one side of the body) in the hands and arms and legs and feet are usually one of the first symptoms observed. Tactile and other fine motor skills are reduced, and often this is most pronounced in handwriting that progressively becomes smaller and less legible. Drawing, needlework, keyboarding, twisting container caps, use of hand tools, and dozens of other routine daily activities also are impaired.

Trouble with gait, posture, and balance are additional prominent and visible symptoms. People with Parkinson's often shuffle their feet as they walk with short strides and bent posture. As the disease progresses some individuals will experience slowness of body motion, referred to as "bradykinesias" or even "freezing", which is temporary paralysis of movement causing the feet to seem to be stuck to the floor. Decline in balance and coordination increases the risk of falling and is especially troublesome for older individuals.

"Dyskinesias," frequently associated with the body's reaction to medications, especially levodopa, includes involuntary exaggerated movements of arms, legs, trunk, neck, and face (think Michael J. Fox). Another impairment, called "dystonia," is caused by muscle contraction that results in abnormal positioning of feet, hands, and toes.

Cognitive and mental disorders related to Parkinson's are especially severe. Memory loss and decline of cognitive ability, "bradyphrenia," impacts an individual's ability to converse effectively, interact appropriately in social settings, and handle multiple priorities. Dementia is a particularly debilitating mental disorder. It is estimated that approximately one-third of Parkinson's patients will experience mild to severe symptoms.

Disabilities related to the autonomic nervous system are less noticeable but significant. Voice and speech disorders, including drooling and voice volume and quality, are common. These disorders make it difficult for Parkinson's patients to be heard and understood. The inability to use facial expression, referred to as "masked face," further inhibits one's ability to communicate. Difficulty digesting food and reflux necessitate changes in diet and timing of meals. "Aspiration," the passage of food or liquid into the lungs, and "dysphagia," impaired swallowing, are serious problems that can in extreme circumstances cause death. Incontinence and constipation are frustrating and sometimes embarrassing Parkinson's symptoms related to the autonomic nervous system and Parkinson's disease.

Depression is an outcome that often goes unrecognized and can significantly affect quality of life.

A majority of people with Parkinson's will experience some degree of depression, especially as the severity of their symptoms increase. Stress and chronic fatigue impair patients' ability to sustain physical and emotional energy. These are underlying but significant disabilities that contribute to depression and exacerbate many other disabilities.

What a lengthy litany of egregious symptoms! And there is no silver bullet or magical medical elixir for eliminating the devastating consequences of Parkinson's. But neither is there cause for despair.

Throughout this book we will accompany you on your journey, sharing information and suggestions to help you live *Parkinson Positive*.

We will challenge you to live courageously each day, doing what you can and managing what you can't.

Medications and medical procedures prescribed and monitored by your neurologist are essential to living positively and productively. They are the foundation on which you will build your plan to combat Parkinson's. Information on the medical treatment of Parkinson's will be covered in chapter five.

You will need a team of health care professionals to help you implement your plan to live *Parkinson Positive*. In the next chapter we will discuss how to assemble and engage your team members.

NUGGETS

- Early diagnosis and intervention are critical. Parkinson's disease is progressive and has reached an advanced stage even before its first symptoms are detected.

- Knowledge is powerful medicine. Educating yourself about Parkinson's—its symptoms and treatment protocols—will enable you to more effectively communicate with your neurologist and health care team members to develop and monitor your treatment plan.

- Medications and medical procedures prescribed and monitored by your neurologist are essential to living positively and productively. They are the foundation on which you will build your plan to combat Parkinson's.

CHAPTER 2

Partners for the Journey

None of us is as smart as all of us.

—KEN BLANCHARD

Reeling from their fresh diagnosis, John and Mary drove home in silence. That evening after dinner, Mary broke the silence. "How do we know if you really have Parkinson's disease? Is this the kind of thing that requires a second opinion?"

"I don't know," John answered slowly. I'm not even sure what kind of doctor I need to see. Our family doctor mentioned neurologists and movement disorder specialists, but I just don't know."

"Well, I know a few things, John," Mary assured. "I love you and we're in this together and we're going to keep asking questions until we understand the answers."

With watery eyes, they embraced and held each other more tightly than they had in years.

Partners for the Journey

As our family (Bruce) has lived with my wife's chronic condition for almost 11 years now, we have learned that we need trusted partners for the journey. Prior to this, we only viewed health professionals as temporary stops on our way back to normal life. But years of living with a chronic condition reshaped our perspective.

We need a team. So do you.

Why? First of all, your team reminds you that you are not alone. When you surround yourself with doctors, friends, family, therapists, support groups, and others, you tend to generate a sense of common purpose, shared experience, and genuine relationship.

Also, you need a team to help with what you do not know or cannot do for yourself. And that's okay. In fact, partnering with other people is a display of intelligence. In most arenas of life, success requires more than one person. For instance, a successful entrepreneur will most likely need marketing, accounting, or management expertise from someone else. Your experience with Parkinson's disease is similar. By surrounding yourself with a team of people with various expertise and contributions, you will optimize your life with PD.

Therefore, you need a team to help you develop a game plan that aligns with your values. For example, your values related to PD may include:

- Maximizing your independence

- Maintaining relationships with family and friends

- Continuing your work or hobbies

- Ensuring your emotional well-being

- Maintaining your activities of daily living

- Managing troublesome side effects

- Reducing your PD symptoms

So, who might be on your team? While the available resources may vary depending on where you live, your team will probably include your primary care physician, your neurologist, and your caregiver. In addition, you may have a nurse, physical therapist, occupational therapist, speech therapist, pharmacist, or mental health professional. Perhaps you are also thinking of friends, family members, and support groups.

You are looking for partners. With a blend of intention and persistence, you will find them. Gail Sheehy, author of *Passages in Caregiving,* describes this well.

> "Partner—that was the word we were looking for."

> Between doctor and patient and caregiver, treatment must be a collaborative process. It is essential that you as caregiver speak up, and right from the start assess whether or not this is a doctor willing to enter into a collaboration."

As you think about the partners and members of your team, you may begin by finding a neurologist.

How to Find a Neurologist

The question before the question is, "Why do I need to see a neurologist? Wouldn't my family doctor be good enough?"

Think of it this way: the specialist specializes. While a general practitioner may see some Parkinson cases each year, a neurologist who focuses on Parkinson's disease may see hundreds of cases each year. Just as you would prefer to take golf lessons from a golf pro, rather than a general athlete who plays golf well, so we recommend that you partner with a neurologist. If possible, we recommend a movement disorder specialist. This is a neurologist who has completed a movement disorder fellowship.

As Malcolm Gladwell describes in *Blink*, the more educated and experienced a person becomes in their field of specialty, the more quickly and accurately they can assess a situation.

Now, you should know that not all neurologists focus on Parkinson patients. Some specialize in MS, brain injury, etc. So, follow these guidelines:

1. Ask around. In particular, call to ask your state or regional Parkinson organization. Ask your friends, if you know someone who shares your diagnosis.

2. Ask your general practitioner for a referral. In some cases, a referral may be required by your insurance anyway. If your general practitioner (GP) or family doctor resists, keep asking.

To begin, you may want to consider these additional questions from Assist Guide Information Services. You might also check the "Selecting a Physician" worksheet in the appendix.

1. Is the doctor in your loved one's insurance company's network of providers?

2. If not, can you or your loved one afford to pay the costs not covered by the insurance company?

3. How much travel time will be required for doctor visits?

4. Does the doctor take an active interest in your loved one's health?

5. Is the doctor receptive to questions?

How to Talk to Your Doctor

As you well know, your time with a doctor is typically limited. Sometimes severely limited! Therefore,

The more prepared you are prior to the visit, the better.

Before your visit, think through the routine of questions that your doctor is likely to ask you and prepare your answers. Be sure to write down three questions that you have as well.

Let her know about changes in symptoms or concerns about sleep patterns, anxiety, or any other developments. Ask about new therapies. Repeat back what the doctor has recommended to ensure clarity.

Some patients find it helpful to maintain a Parkinson's journal or binder to keep up with medications, symptoms, questions, and other developments. Whether this takes a written or digital form, you might consider some type of system to stay organized and prepared.

To optimize your communication with your doctor, you might consider some of these questions:

- What does my doctor need to hear from me?

- How can I give the most accurate picture of my symptoms?

- Which daily activities are most important? Enlist your doctor to help you do what you want to be able to keep doing.

Parkinson Organization

Jerry and I partner with the Parkinson Foundation of Oklahoma. Throughout this book, you may find references to a few national Parkinson groups as well as a few regional organizations. But, you should have some level of access to a group near you.

Each group offers a different variety of services. For instance, the Parkinson Foundation of Oklahoma focuses on these programs:

- Support groups

- Exercise groups

- Education conferences

- SPEAK OUT® voice therapy and subsequent LOUD Crowd® groups to maintain swallowing muscles and voice volume

- Family consultations

- Parkinson's 101 classes

- Special educational events on a variety of timely topics

Look up Parkinson organizations with a presence in your state or surrounding states. Take advantage of educational or exercise programs.

Connect with other Parkinson families near you.

Your team is incomplete without some ties to a local Parkinson organization.

Physical Therapist or Exercise Classes

Ask your local Parkinson organization about PD specific physical therapy or exercise options in your area. According to the Parkinson's Disease Clinic and Research Center in San Francisco,

> *"Regular exercise benefits people with Parkinson's disease.*

Exercise reduces stiffness and improves mobility, posture, balance and gait." Be sure to ask about physical therapists who have experience treating people with a neurological disorder, and specifically with PD.

You will also want to inquire about Parkinson specific exercise classes in your area. Many organizations offer Tai Chi, Yoga, dance, non-contact boxing, or other exercise classes for PD patients. Becky Farley has developed the PWR! (Parkinson Wellness Recovery) programs that are offered by trained Physical Therapists around the country, often through hospitals and clinics. In fact, Jerry has completed this program and found it to be quite helpful with balance, gait, and flexibility.

A multitude of exercise books and routines exist, but the crucial move is to begin and to continue exercising. Whether alone, with friends, through a class, or as a physical therapy program, we urge you to exercise!

Voice Therapist

Secondary symptoms of PD may include dysphagia (swallowing difficulty) and softness of voice. The Parkinson Voice Project based in Richardson, Texas has developed an innovative therapy to improve swallowing and voice volume. Also, the Lee Silverman Voice Therapy (LSVT) program trains clinicians in similar ways.

Did you know that researchers estimate that 89% of Parkinson's patients will experience speech and voice impairment? Professor Ramig and her colleagues from the University of Colorado have led the way in signaling the call for intensive voice treatment in Parkinson's patients. Currently, however, a very small percentage of PD patients engage in treatment.

According to Samantha Elandary of the Parkinson Voice Project, "It is possible to save a voice that appears to be deteriorating as a result of this neurodegenerative condition." Elandary goes on to say, "Traditional speech therapy does not work with Parkinson's...The key is early intervention—the sooner patients enroll in voice therapy, the better their chances to regain the strength of their voices."

With intentional guided exercise of those muscles, you should expect improvement. And, maintenance exercise certainly increases the chances of sustaining your improvements for as long as possible.

Other Help

Since the food we eat plays an important role in our health and wellbeing, you may find it helpful to consult with a nutritionist. If you have had PD for very long, you have probably been sold all types of magical cures for your disease. While we doubt that there really is a "magic bullet" out there, we do encourage you to incorporate a healthy diet into your plan.

A nutritionist can help you determine the best priorities of foods for your body. Taking into account your PD, as well as any other conditions, a nutritionist will consider your medications and help you develop a healthy eating plan to support better quality of life.

Another source of help could be an occupational therapist. According to the Parkinson Disease Foundation, "Occupational Therapy (OT) may be able to help people with PD more effectively perform everyday activities such as self-care and household chores."

An occupational therapist can help you with treatment and recommendations for a wide variety of daily activities such as handwriting, driving evaluation, cooking, eating, computer modifications, and more. Ask your doctor if OT might be helpful for you.

Licensed Professional Counselor

According to an article by Irene Richard and Roger Kurlan on the under-recognition of depression in Parkinson's, "about 50% of patients with PD experience depression. Recent evidence indicates that depression is the major factor negatively affecting quality of life in PD and that emotional symptoms, including depression, are the main cause of caregiver distress. Thus, effective treatment of co-morbid depression has the potential of improving overall function and quality of life for both patients and caregivers."

If you or your caree are experiencing symptoms such as a sense of helplessness or hopelessness, anger, loss of interest in daily activities, or changes in sleep, appetite, or energy, ask for help.

Many health insurance plans now cover a limited number of therapy visits. Or, you may want to utilize an employer's EAP (Employee Assistance Program) or research subsidized counseling for caregivers in your area. Through one of these avenues there are people who can help guide you.

Inviting good team members to partner with you is crucial. But in order to be a good team member yourself, you will need to understand how to help others help you. The next chapter will equip you to do this!

NUGGETS

- It is imperative to select a neurologist who has experience working with Parkinson's patients. Moreover, you should trust and feel comfortable working with your neurologist.

- You also will need to put together a team of health care professionals to help you develop a plan customized to treat your Parkinson's symptoms and meet your personal needs. Your team might include a physical therapist, occupational therapist, voice therapist, nutritionist, pharmacist, or mental health professional.

- Prepare in advance for each visit with your neurologist. He or she will have limited time to visit with you, and you will need to maximize the benefits of each appointment. Write down the questions you want to ask your doctor, and provide him or her with a list of your responses to medications and changes in your symptoms since your last appointment.

CHAPTER 3

Helping Others Help You

Courage is the finest of human qualities
because it guarantees all the others.
—WINSTON CHURCHILL

"I don't want to ask for help," he stated rather bluntly. *"I don't want pity either."*

"Neither do I, Honey. But, we don't know it all and we can't do it all. The truth is that we need some help to understand this disease and we need some help to live well with it," she replied.

Silence.

But within that silence, he knew she was right. And with that, they agreed to begin helping others help them.

Telling Other People

Telling other people about your Parkinson's causes feelings of vulnerability. As Brene Brown describes in her book, *Daring Greatly,* "Vulnerability isn't good or bad: It's not what we call a dark emotion, nor is it always a light, positive experience. Vulnerability is the core of all emotions and feelings. To feel is to be vulnerable."

No doubt, PD gives rise to anxiety and fear... at least a little bit. *What happens next? What if I fall? How quickly will it progress? What if people judge me unfairly or are afraid of me? Will I lose my job? What if people withdraw or just don't understand?*

If you experienced any hesitation in sharing your new diagnosis with family members, you are completely normal! But be careful not to confuse vulnerability or feelings of uncertainty with weakness.

Neither breaking the news to family members, nor seeking wise counsel from a neurologist or other health professional shows signs of weakness. Vulnerable? Yes. Weakness? No.

"Vulnerability sounds like truth and feels like courage.

Truth and courage aren't always comfortable, but they're never weakness," asserts Brene Brown.

Breaking the News

So, how do you break the news? How do you tell your story? Over time, you may get better and better at your telling. In the beginning, you may not have much to say. Still, you want to say it as well as you can. To begin, consider these guidelines and invest the time to rehearse and practice what you will say.

- List three to seven significant points or moments along your way thus far. You may think of early symptoms and suspicions, deciding to see a doctor, the day of diagnosis, initial fears, current plans for managing PD, and resources of hope discovered thus far.

- What is the point? If you could only speak one sentence to help someone understand, what would you say?

- Consider what they can do and be prepared to give them some direction. For instance, you may suggest that they attend a PD conference or meeting with you to learn more. Or, you may suggest future possibilities, but simply ask them to stand by you and learn with you for now.

Some of the PD patients we know, have said things such as:

- "I may have Parkinson's, but Parkinson's doesn't have me!"

- "Parkinson's may be a life sentence at this point in time, but it isn't a death sentence."

- "This is not what I planned on, but I have faced adversity before and we will find a way to live the best that we can."

Initially, the new language of medicines and symptoms can be disorienting and overwhelming. For this reason, it is crucial that you connect with people who can help. Ask questions, learn, and listen to people who have been living with PD for a while. As weeks turn into months, you may find that your anxiety decreases in direct inverse proportion to your increase in support and knowledge.

Where once you could see little hope, you now begin to see possibilities for living well with Parkinson's disease. As your understanding advances, hope will seem less cliché and more concrete.

Therefore, revise your story as you go along to incorporate more and more hope and gratitude. The people who hear your story need that desperately.

Refining Your Story

Why this language of "telling your story?" Whether you are the type of person who is inclined to share your story or not, people will ask. You will be put on the spot, and your reply will be much better if you have thought about it ahead of time.

But, who will ask? Your grandchild might ask why your hand shakes. The waitress may notice you spilling your food and put you on the spot. Sitting in the doctor's office waiting area, a fellow patient might inquire about how long you've had PD. You don't always invite the questions, but when you are prepared, your explanations will be better in these unexpected moments.

As you grapple with the disorientation of a new diagnosis, you may tend to slip into the "victim mentality." To regain a fuller perspective, consider your experience thus far from the template of:

- Challenge

- Choices

- Outcomes

Both motor symptoms and non-motor symptoms may make the list. Tremors, stiffness, and how these manifest in particular situations could be part of your challenge. So first, define your **challenges.**

Remember to identify non-motor challenges as well. If you have experienced depression, frustration, or anger, articulate how these emotions have impacted your life. Perhaps you would include sleeplessness, gastro-intestinal issues, and early fatigue, both physical and mental.

Next, think back to the **choices** you made or are making. You may have chosen to engage in a PD specific therapy. Perhaps you talked with a counselor, or instituted some new habits and rhythms into your life to combat the challenges you experienced. What choices did you make in response to the challenges that came your way?

Finally, consider the **outcomes**. Have any of these choices resulted in improvement in any way? Even slight improvement counts. The goal is progress, not perfection.

By defining your experience through this template, you may realize several benefits. First of all, these questions force you into an expectant posture of action. You will not sit idly by, while the disease runs its course. Instead, by responding to your challenges with choices, you expect better outcomes.

Furthermore, clarity may emerge. Sometimes the right question helps us cut through the fog to place our finger on the pulse of the problem or the solution.

Besides benefitting you, as you learn to assess and tell your story through the lens of this template, other people may benefit from your model.

Understanding Yourself and Others

"Everybody's weird." On multiple occasions, I heard a former boss make this declaration. His tone was neither judgmental nor condescending. Simply put, these words reminded us that each of our clients and co-workers are unique individuals, complete with idiosyncrasies, charming hallmarks, and frustrating tendencies.

"Everybody's weird."

So are you.

So am I.

But what good does this do us? Basically, a growing sense of self-awareness helps us become more gracious with ourselves and others. If you have some understanding of your personality type, conflict style, family system and more, you will probably be more comfortable in your own skin and less defensive about your flaws. You may even give other people some slack.

Personality Types

Some of us renew our energy by being around people, while the rest of us need solitude to refuel our engines. As newlyweds, my wife and I discovered this difference. When I arrived home from work each day, I immediately went to sit on the balcony of our small apartment to breathe, stare at the trees, and decompress. After about 15-30 minutes, I was ready and happy to see my wife.

What I didn't know until the second year of our marriage was that while I sat on the balcony, my wife worried that I didn't like her! She wanted to talk and share details of the day and basically be together. This is how she found renewal from the day.

As it turns out, there is nothing wrong with either one of us. We simply have opposite tendencies in this regard.

For instance, an extroverted, light-hearted person may choose to host a dinner party to break the news and solicit the encouragement of friends and family. Quite differently, an introverted, detail oriented person may decide to be very careful and specific about how much information is given to whom and under what circumstances.

Volumes of good books and helpful tools are awaiting you, if you determine that you need to learn more about personality types. For our purposes, if you are going to help others help you, you will do well to have some understanding about yourself and others and the dynamics that make us all tick.

Conflict Styles

Another inevitable, but often overlooked, facet of understanding ourselves and others concerns our conflict styles.

Conflict is not inherently bad, but the way we handle it can be.

Some of us avoid any friction whatsoever, while others of us kick into attack mode at the slightest provocation. Neither extreme proves particularly useful. But the tendencies remain. With heightened self-awareness and new skill learning, we can consciously alter how we handle conflict.

We may even develop the skill to become effective peacemakers and negotiators for mutually beneficial solutions in our family care settings.

For now, just consider that people respond to and process conflict differently. Ask yourself, *How does your typical response and handling of conflict affect your situation for good or ill?*

Does this diagnosis of Parkinson's make you mad or sad or both?

Are you more likely to excuse slights or misunderstandings or are you more inclined to explode in anger?

To a certain extent, these are both natural responses to conflict and problems. However, you must know that extreme avoidance or anger typically do more harm than good.

Therefore, PD patients who become aware of their conflict tendencies and work to respond peaceably tend to generate energy around them that is helpful not harmful.

Family Systems

No person is an island unto himself. Essentially, this forms an armchair definition of family systems theory. When Dad is diagnosed with Parkinson's, it's not just his problem. This new reality will change life for Mom, as well as for the children and maybe even siblings and friends. Attempts at isolation are typically not helpful. Acknowledge the realities of your disease, and intentionally seek to include your family in the process and challenge of living optimally nevertheless.

By inviting help, you create space for expressions of love and caring and courage. Your family needs you to allow them to be a part of the solution.

Perhaps these brief reminders will prompt you to recollect or dig out data from previously taken personality inventories or peruse helpful notes or books from your recent past. Or, maybe this nudge will move you into new discovery with the tools recommended.

But at a minimum, please take a moment to reflect on what makes you and the people in your life tick. Withhold unnecessary judgment and simply attune your senses to the beauty of the uniqueness of each person. Perhaps it won't be that simple. Still, consider appreciating what you cannot control. And move back into reality with a bit more grace for yourself and others.

Educating Others

Besides merely telling your story, you may find that you need to educate others about Parkinson's disease. You can safely assume that you know more than most of your friends and family. First-hand experience deals its share of problems, but it also gives you a high degree of credibility. Still, it is crucial that you, the patient, continue to educate yourself. As you learn more, you stay up-to-date with the latest treatments, insights, and options.

Egregious assumptions abound. For instance, try not to be too offended if someone thinks PD is contagious. In fact, you might become an expert in reframing conversations as you hear any number of faulty ideas about PD.

Be patient. Explain the realities of PD.

Guide your friends and family into a better understanding.

Since some symptoms are more noticeable than others, you might start there and practice your answers to these questions to be prepared to educate others.

Now that you're forming your team and helping others help you, let's talk about how they can help you with your activities of daily living. Join us in chapter four as we address specific coping strategies for what you want to be able to do.

NUGGETS

- Parkinson's is not just your disease; it impacts your family and friends as well. Newly diagnosed with Parkinson's, you will feel vulnerable and perhaps for the first time a sense of inadequacy. You may be afraid that others will now view you differently, and you will be anxious about how to explain this disease. These are normal fears that most people with Parkinson's initially experience.

- An important step in coming to terms with Parkinson's is learning how to help others help you. Family, friends, and colleagues you work with and who care about you will want to understand your Parkinson's disabilities and how they can best support you. You have an opportunity to transform this circle of family and friends into a knowledgeable, caring support team.

CHAPTER 4

Coping Strategies

When one door closes another door opens; but we so often look so long and regretfully upon the closed door, that we do not see the ones that open for us.
—ALEXANDER GRAHAM BELL

Social embarrassment loomed heavily once again. With most of his symptoms under reasonable control, he returned to the Rotary Club meeting. Smiles and pats on the back welcomed him, but as he scanned the room, he spotted trouble: the lunch line.

Sure, the caterers would serve the food, but he would have to carry a plate and cup to the table. Not wanting to ask for help, he made two trips. But still, his tremors caused him to spill a noticeable amount of his drink before he could get to the table.

How, he wondered, could he manage this any better?

Challenges and solutions. In this chapter, we will expose some of the most daunting, daily tests in what used to be normal routines. Perhaps you will discover some tools, tricks, or practical ideas to simplify your daily living experiences.

Clothing and Dressing

One of your first challenges each morning and one of the last each evening arrives as you attempt to get dressed. Shoelaces, buttons, zippers, as well as the flexibility and balance to place legs and arms in their respective places pose significant problems.

First of all, be sure to allow ample time. Granted, your mind may still default to the routine amount of time it took to get ready for decades. But now, you require more time. Allow for it.

Set realistic expectations.

Your frustration level may begin to decline.

Consider the order of your morning routine. How much time does your medicine require to take effect? How can you best order medicine, breakfast, bathing, and dressing for optimal results?

For difficult clothing maneuvers related to zippers, you might try a ring-pull device. For pants and stockings, you may need someone to help. Or, you could use a sock-pulling tool. For shoes, you can purchase or create a long-handled shoehorn.

Did you know that numerous companies cater to these specific needs? You can learn more by contacting one of these companies or locate your own source for clothing designed for Parkinson patients.

- buckandbuck.com

- Silverts.com

- magnaready.com

Eating and Dining Out

As the vignette at the beginning of this chapter illustrated, dining in public can be difficult. In fact, as the disease progresses, eating at all can prove vexing.

The European Parkinson Disease Association states, "Most people with Parkinson's experience dysphagia due to the reduced control they have of their mouth and throat muscles, especially in the later stages of the condition. Eating becomes slower, more hesitant and requires more effort. It can become increasingly difficult to clear the mouth of saliva, and to swallow instinctively when muscles become weak or rigid."

Innovative programs such as the Parkinson Voice Project can help build the muscles that contribute to more efficient swallowing as well as louder speaking volume. In most cases, this therapy requires an initial intensive program of several weeks followed by a maintenance regimen of daily or weekly exercises.

According to the National Parkinson Foundation, these general tips will get you started in the right direction:

- Schedule meals during "on" times, or when medication is working best.

- Cut food into small bite-size pieces so that it is easier to chew and swallow.

- If you have swallowing problems, don't drink thin liquids or use a straw.

- Sit up as straight as possible when eating, and stay upright for at least 30 minutes after each meal.

For eating at home, a number of assistive devices are available that can minimize frustration and maximize quality of life. For example, spill proof cups as well as cups that eliminate the need to tilt your head back can be helpful. Or, you might find that rocker knives, utensils with oversized handles, or scoop plates make mealtime less messy. In recent years, counter balancing, self-stabilizing spoons, such as the one from Liftware, are becoming more common for patients with tremors.

Personal Hygiene

For the Parkinson patient, the bathroom can often become a dangerous place. Fortunately, bathroom aids have become plentiful in recent years. Have you considered the use of a shower chair, or installing grab bars?

As in all rooms of the house, the Parkinson family needs to be prudent about clearing the clutter and removing rugs that increase the chances of tripping.

According to the Aged Carer, these tips may be helpful:

- Installing grab rails in and outside the shower recess to increase stability and protect against slips and falls

- Using a stable shower seat to sit on whilst showering with a hand held hose

- Place rubber mats on slippery tiles

- Use an electric toothbrush for brushing teeth

- Attach soft grip handles to brushes and combs

- Use soap on tap to avoid soap residue in the shower

- Use an electric razor

- Gather all equipment before you begin

- Ensure someone is wearing his or her medical alarm pendant

- Use a raised toilet seat to ease transferring on and off a toilet

Sleeping

Ahhh, a good night's sleep. Remember those? If you have lived with PD for very long, you have most likely experienced trouble resting at night.

According to the Parkinson Disease Foundation, "Rigid muscles, tremors or stiffness at night, or not being able to roll over in bed can all interfere with sleep, as can the frequent urge to urinate. In addition, many people with Parkinson's experience vivid dreams or hallucinations and act out their dreams, violent nightmares, a problem called 'REM sleep behavior disorder'."

So, what can you do to rest better at night? The Sleep Foundation offers the following suggestions:

- Keep a regular sleep schedule, going to bed and getting up at the same time each day.

- Take sedating medication late enough in the day so that you don't get an increase in symptoms as you are trying to sleep.

- Use satin sheets and pajamas to help with getting in and out of bed.

- Minimize beverages before bedtime to help avoid nocturia (frequent nighttime urination).

- Get exercise and exposure to light early in the day.

Naturally, you will want to discuss your specific situation with your doctor. Still, you may find that some of these suggestions lead to a better night's sleep.

Walking

One of the first things PD patients notice is a change in their gait. With rigidity and a growing sense of imbalance come smaller steps and a more protective walk.

According to a seminal study in 1994 by four researchers in Australia, "Gait hypokinesia (slowness) is a characteristic feature of Parkinson's disease. It is not clear, however, whether the slowness is due to a problem in regulation of the timing of consecutive steps or the control of stride size. The findings indicated that cadence control remains unaffected throughout its entire range in Parkinson's disease and that gait hypokinesia is directly attributable to an inability to internally generate sufficiently large steps." This conclusion begs the question of how the brain and body can be engaged.

In 2011, a research project led by Dr. Anat Mirleman experimented with twenty patients using a combination of treadmill training and virtual reality. They concluded that this therapy, "is viable in PD and may significantly improve physical performance, gait during complex challenging conditions, and even certain aspects of cognitive function. These findings have important implications for understanding motor learning in the presence of PD and for treating fall risk in PD, aging, and others who share a heightened risk of falls."

Becky Farley, the founder of PWR! (Parkinson Wellness Recovery) offers an aggressive exercise therapy program that emphasizes large, exaggerated movements. Farley and Hirsch note that studies suggest, "Exercise may promote brain repair and reorganization (neuroplasticity) in people with PD."

Intentional exercise remains an essential component of better walking.

If your condition declines, however, you may need to consider these helpful tips to make walking easier and safer:

- Use mental or auditory cues to remind yourself to take "big steps" or "long steps."

- Remove throw rugs and clear away obstacles in the home to reduce the chance for falls.

- Create wide pathways in the home wherever possible.

- Take special care with thresholds; perhaps even consider reflective tape in these areas.

Managing Depression

As mentioned earlier in chapter two, half of Parkinson patients will experience some level of clinical depression. Typically, when we become depressed, we eat too much and exercise too little. As feelings of despair squeeze out better thoughts, patients tend to neglect the best practices of self-care in favor of choices that ultimately create a downward spiral.

Therefore, we encourage you to acknowledge and address your depression sooner than later. The earlier you face this bitter reality, and ask for help, the better. Utilize your Employee Assistance Program, health insurance, or other local resources to connect with a trained Licensed Professional Counselor.

Depending on the severity of your experience, a counselor or therapist may suggest a wide array of tools and exercises to help your best self re-emerge. Most likely, you will find that a toolbox full of new ideas, practices, and habits will equip you to cope better.

Simply talking to a neutral third party often provides a release valve for pent up concerns and worries. You can do this! Do not be ashamed. Depression affects many people, and many people have found their way out with the guidance of trained counselors.

As Dr. Leslie Frazier posits, "Coping…is crucial for managing cognitive and psychosocial changes associated with illness. Coping effectively may be the buffer that preserves quality of life."

As you implement these coping strategies for daily living, medications will also play a crucial role. Turn to chapter five to learn more about the medications and medical procedures that can improve your life with PD.

NUGGETS

- As the symptoms of Parkinson's increase in severity, you will need to implement strategies to accommodate the attendant challenges.

- You can continue to experience quality life and be socially active, if you are willing to adapt and to initiate life skills to overcome these challenges.

- There are practical tools and techniques to help you with clothing, dressing yourself, eating, personal hygiene and other daily necessities and to help you be more comfortable in social situations.

CHAPTER 5

Medications and Medical Procedures

Whether you think you can, or think you can't…
you're right.

—HENRY FORD

"**I** don't think this medicine is working," John vented. "That guy in the exercise group is taking the same dose I am and I never see his tremors."

"Remember, John, Parkinson's is unique to each person. Let's add this to the list to ask the neurologist about at our visit next week," Mary said calmly.

"You're right," John agreed. "But until we get the tremors under control, it's still frustrating."

Understanding Medical Treatments

Developing and managing your medication plan is the most important element of living positively with Parkinson's.

Having a basic understanding of drugs prescribed for Parkinson's will help you more effectively partner with doctors and other health care professionals on your team. This knowledge, coupled with information about the symptoms of Parkinson's covered in chapter one, will enable you to work with your doctor to assess and adjust your medication needs and treatment as you transition through progressive stages of Parkinson's. The risk of overwhelming you with information overload is worth the potential benefit of empowering you to be proactive in managing your Parkinson's medication protocol.

It is our intent to provide you with information on drugs that will be both informative and yet readily understandable. Persons seeking a comprehensive and scholarly examination of Parkinson's medications and medical procedures will be directed to publications listed in the Recommended Resources.. The following review is not intended to offer medical advice or make any claims about the appropriateness or effectiveness of any medication or medical procedure.

Individuals should consult with their doctor before making any decisions about managing their medication protocol.

As has been noted, Parkinson's is progressive. And to date, there are no proven drugs, therapies, or medical procedures that will cure this disease or even significantly slow its progression, though there are conflicting claims. But medications currently available for Parkinson's treatment can lessen the severity of your symptoms and help you live a productive and meaningful life, often for many years, after you have been diagnosed.

"We emphasize that knowledge is powerful medicine."

We will provide you with an overview of four groups of medications most frequently prescribed for Parkinson's patients. And we will point out potential benefits and risks of these drugs and the intervention role each plays in the treatment of Parkinson's.

Medications for Treating Parkinson's

Different individuals respond differently to similar drugs.

As you progress through the stages of Parkinson's, you will need to work with your neurologist to help modify your medication plan. This includes different doses, timing of dosages, and adding or dropping drugs. A cautionary note: do not deviate from your plan without first consulting with your doctor. Developing a personalized medication plan appropriate to your needs can be daunting. Having a basic understanding of commonly prescribed drugs and medical procedures can help you be more proactive, positive, and confident in developing the right plan for you.

As previously discussed, Parkinson's disease is caused by a critical decline of dopamine in the brain—up to 80% before symptoms are observable.

The fundamental challenge, then, for treating Parkinson's is to administer medications that will increase the amount of dopamine in the brain or replace dopamine that has been lost.

But dopamine administered orally or by injection does not directly enter the brain because it cannot pass the blood-brain barrier. This barrier is a network of blood vessels that filters blood flowing into the brain and blocks certain substances, including dopamine, from entering.

Levodopa And Carbidopa

Levodopa is the most effective and commonly prescribed drug for enabling the replenishment of dopamine in the brain. Levodopa is a type of amino acid and precursor to dopamine. It can pass the blood-brain barrier and enter the brain. It is then converted into dopamine by action of the enzyme "dopa decarboxylase."

Levodopa has been prescribed since the 1960s. It appropriately has been referred to as the "gold standard" for the treatment of Parkinson's disease.

And it will be the foundational medication for treatment of your Parkinson's symptoms.

Levodopa helps treat disabilities commonly associated with Parkinson's. These include tremors, bradykenesia (slowness of movement), motor function and balance, memory loss, hypomemia (masked face), and dystonia (a muscle contraction state, resulting in abnormal positioning of feet, toes, hand, and other body parts). Studies have substantiated that many people with Parkinson's can function relatively well for many years with levodopa treatment in conjunction with other medications and health care interventions.

Unfortunately, as Parkinson's progresses and increasingly stronger and more frequent doses are prescribed, levodopa often becomes less effective (referred to as "wearing off"). Another concern is that the cumulative effect of increased daily dosage of levodopa and other drugs potentially can increase the risk of developing dyskinesia (involuntary, uncontrollable movement of head and limbs).

However, there is continuing debate and differing opinions about the risk of dyskinesia caused by extensive use of levodopa. Levodopa may also contribute to motor fluctuations, the "on-off" effect (cyclic periods of drug working and not working), gait, and freezing (inability to move feet and limbs). The degree of risk of developing these symptoms is currently being reconsidered and debated by researchers. Many neurologists feel that the early benefits of levodopa to the quality of life of patients outweigh any potential long-term risks that they might incur.

Carbidopa does not directly treat symptoms of Parkinson's. However, it is important because it helps block the conversion of levodopa to dopamine while it is in the circulatory system. As mentioned earlier, dopamine cannot cross the blood-brain barrier. Carbidopa enables more levodopa to reach the brain and be converted to dopamine. It also helps reduce nausea often associated with levodopa. Levodopa is prescribed in combination with the drug carbidopa, under the brand name, Sinemet, or as a generic. When referring to this drug and other formulations as "levodopa," which is common practice, it is understood to include both carbidopa and levodopa.

There are two major formulations of levodopa—"immediate release" and "sustained release."

Regular levodopa (immediate release) is usually prescribed in three tablet dosages: 25-100, 10-100, and 25-250. These numbers refer to milligrams--the first is carbidopa and the second levodopa. Sustained release formulations include: Sinemet CR (controlled-release), Sinemet SR (sustained-release), and Paracopa (extended release). Immediate release levodopa will get into the system nearly twice as fast (approximately 30 to 45 minutes) as controlled release. But its effectiveness will start to decline after two hours. Controlled release formulations generally last a couple of hours longer.

In January of 2015, The U.S. Food and Drug Administration (FDA) approved "RYTARY" for the treatment of Parkinson's. RYTARY is an oral capsule formulation of levodopa that contains both immediate and extended release beads (1:4 carbidopa-levodopa ratio of beads). Its purpose is to reduce the amount of "off time" experienced by Parkinson's patients, especially those in advanced stages. It is offered in four strengths. Parkinson's patients should not use RYTARY if they are taking a nonselective monoamine oxidase (MAO) inhibitor.

The FDA also approved, in January 2015, "DUOPA" for use in patients with advanced Parkinson's who are experiencing increasing motor fluctuations and off time. DUOPA is an enteral suspension of carbidopa-levodopa administered through a tube inserted into the small intestine by a small infusion pump. This procedure bypasses the stomach and delivers carbidopa and levodopa directly into the small intestine. There are risks, including stomach blockage and infection, associated with this procedure. It should not be taken by patients who also are using a nonselective monoamine oxidase (MAO) inhibitor.

Physicians often will start a Parkinson's patient in the initial or early stages with immediate release carbidopa-levodopa. The most commonly prescribed dosage will be the 25-100 tablet, three to four times daily, equally spaced throughout the day. As Parkinson's disease progresses, it likely will be necessary to increase the dosage or the frequency of taking the tablets to maintain optimal benefits of levodopa to the patient. Additional drugs will be added later to the medication plan, as needed.

It is important to note that for optimum results, levodopa administered orally should be taken on an empty stomach (at least one hour before meals or two hours following meals). Dietary protein in the stomach can interfere with the absorption of levodopa into the bloodstream and eventually the brain. Vitamin pills that contain iron also can inhibit levodopa from being absorbed and should not be taken at the same time.

Dopamine Agonists

Dopamine agonists are the second most frequently prescribed group of medications used to treat Parkinson's. A dopamine agonist is a synthetic drug that closely resembles the chemical structure of the neurotransmitter dopamine. But unlike dopamine, it can cross the blood-brain barrier, enter the brain, and stimulate dopamine receptors there. Dopamine agonist medications are not as potent as levodopa. They can be used alone or in combination with levodopa to help get more dopamine to the brain.

First generation dopamine agonist drugs include bromocriptine (Paralodel) and pergolide (Permax). Second generation drugs which currently are more commonly prescribed include: pramipexole (Mirapex) and ropinirole (Requip, Requip XL), rotigotine (Neupro) administered by patch, and apomorphine (Apokyn) taken through injection.

An agonist may be the only medication prescribed early in the disease, while the symptoms are still relatively mild. The intent of this strategy is to delay the need for levodopa treatment as long as possible to defer the risks associated with long-term usage. However, a dopamine agonist used alone will not sufficiently control Parkinson's symptoms very long. Most doctors will prescribe levodopa as the initial drug, either by itself or in combination with a dopamine agonist or other drug.

A second purpose for prescribing a dopamine agonist is to help reduce fluctuations in the levodopa response that develop over time. For this reason, agonists are often added later to the medication plan. And finally, some studies suggest that pramipexole and ropinirole help slow the progression of Parkinson's. However, this has not been adequately documented.

These drugs also help diminish nighttime leg cramps and control tremors associated with Parkinson's. Potential risks include: nausea, decrease in blood pressure, hallucinations and paranoia, excessive daytime sleepiness, sudden sleep attacks, personality and behavioral changes, swelling of ankles and feet, and water retention.

Enzyme Inhibitors/Levodopa Extenders

A third group of medications referred to as "enzyme inhibitors" or "levodopa extenders" help block the action of two enzymes that break down and change levodopa in the circulatory system to an ineffective substance before it can reach the brain. These enzymes are catechol-O-methyltransferase (COMT) and monoamine oxidase (MAO). There are two forms of the MAO enzyme—MAO-A and MAO-B. Because of potentially severe side effects, drugs that inhibit MAO-A are seldom prescribed.

COMT inhibitor drugs prescribed for Parkinson's are entacapone (Comtan) and tolcapone (Tasmar). Entacapone, when combined in one pill with carbidopa and levodopa, is sold under the brand name Stalevo. MAO-B inhibitor drugs used for treating Parkinson's are selegiline (Eldepryl) and rasagiline (Azilect).

COMT enzyme inhibitors have no benefit in treating Parkinson's when used alone and require the use of levodopa concurrently. MAO-B inhibitors, however, can have benefit independently and can be used in monotherapy or in conjunction with levodopa.

There are risks associated with taking enzyme inhibitors. They can indirectly contribute to levodopa-induced dyskinesia. Additional risks include: low blood pressure, dizziness, nausea, vomiting, and hallucinations. Tolcapone can also damage the liver.

Anticholinergics

Anticholinergic medications suppress the effects of acetylcholine, a neurotransmitter located in the striatum. They are different from other drugs regularly prescribed for Parkinson's in that they do not act directly on the dopamine system. Trihexyphenidyl (Artane) and benztropine (Cogentin) are prescribed drugs included in this category.

Acetylcholine competes with dopamine in the striatum and diminishes its effectiveness. This is especially true as dopamine levels begin to decline due to Parkinson's. The rationale for anticholinergic drugs is to block the increasing effect of cholinergic cells that release acetylcholine in the striatum.

Anticholinergic medications are sometimes prescribed in the early stages of Parkinson's to help reduce tremors and motor problems, but they are usually ineffective in later stages. These drugs are only moderately effective, and their benefit should be weighed against the potential side effects: blurred vision, constipation, difficulty urinating, muscle cramps, erectile dysfunction, sleepiness, dry mouth, confusion, memory loss, hallucinations, and irritability. For these reasons, anticholinergic drugs are not commonly prescribed.

Managing Your Medications

We have provided information (you may be thinking too much) to help you better understand the benefits and risks of drugs commonly prescribed for Parkinson's. You will be taking multiple medications and different dosages of drugs as you progress through different stages of the disease. Medications used to treat Parkinson's are complex and powerful with potentially severe side effects. To achieve maximum benefit and minimize adverse reactions, they should be used precisely as prescribed by your doctor. And the timing and dosage of medications are critical. Michael Okun in his book, *Parkinson's Treatment: 10 Secrets to A Happier Life*, emphasizes that the, "timing of medication doses is in many cases more important than the dose itself." Carefully administer and monitor your medications.

Do not change dosage or frequency of medications without first consulting with your doctor.

Keep your doctor informed about additional medications (prescription and over-the-counter) that you are taking and talk with him or her before taking any additional drugs, especially antibiotics, pain killers, sleep aids, cold medicine, and dietary supplements.

Your pharmacist can also be an excellent source of information for you, and you may want to consider purchasing all your drugs from one pharmacy. Your pharmacist will have a record of all the prescription drugs you are taking and can help advise you about drug interactions.

She will be able to answer questions you may have and advise you about benefits and possible risks of drugs you are taking. And your pharmacist can make you aware of generic drugs that will cost significantly less than the equivalent branded ones. But before you make any substitutions, first consult your physician.

There is another member of your medication team that you may not have thought about—your health insurance provider. You may be thinking, "The only interaction I have with my insurance company is to haggle over coverage and costs for medications and medical services." We urge you to consider the benefits of a more positive relationship with your insurance provider.

Before you add a new medication or other medical service, consult your insurance coverage plan.

Annually, your insurance provider will send you information on your coverage plan, highlighting updates and changes to your plan. Additionally, you will receive a booklet listing drugs (a "formulary") that are covered by your insurance provider. Another booklet (a "pharmacy directory") will also be mailed to you. It will list pharmacies that are pre-approved by your insurance company. To qualify for drug benefits, you normally will be required to use a pharmacy included in your provider's network.

Read these insurance documents carefully and consult them before you make decisions about adding new medications and services. If you have questions, contact a service representative of your company via its toll free phone number. Representatives are knowledgeable about your coverage, and they can provide information that will assist you in managing your health care plan. You can also ask your pharmacist to assist you in communicating with your insurance provider.

As emphasized in chapter two, this idea will be helpful.

Keep a journal of your responses to medications you are taking and details of the progression of your Parkinson's symptoms.

This will help prepare you to discuss necessary modifications to your medication plan with your doctor and pharmacist. You may want to refer to your journal to help you prepare questions and share insights with your doctor that you might otherwise forget.

Most doctors want feedback from patients and are willing to address their concerns, but their appointment schedules are full, and the time they can spend with any one patient is limited. Knowing in advance what issues and concerns you want to address with your doctor will maximize the effectiveness of your limited time together.

Prepare a list of all your medications and dosage instructions and share a copy with your spouse, family members or other caregiver. You may also want to provide a copy to your primary care physician. Keep a list of your medications and dosage in your wallet or purse for handy reference. For drugs that require multiple daily dosages, levodopa for example, carry pills with you in your pocket or purse to ensure that you take them in a timely manner.

Parkinson's is your disease—own it and manage it.

This will require that you coordinate and complement your medication plan with other health care interventions, including exercise, diet, voice exercises, emotional counseling, and other therapies. Elements of these health care therapies are covered in other chapters.

Medical Procedures

Brain surgery to treat Parkinson's dates back several decades, but positive results have often been negligible and included attendant risks. Research and surgery in recent years has focused on stimulating targeted parts of the brain with low intensity, high frequency electrical current.

Deep brain stimulation (DBS) has emerged as the most effective and widely used surgical procedure for treating Parkinson's.

This two-part procedure involves drilling small dime-sized holes through the skull and implanting electrodes into targeted areas of the brain. In follow-up surgery, a battery-powered neurostimulator device is connected by a wire under the skin to the electrode and implanted in the chest, much like a pacemaker for the heart. It sends electrical pulses to areas of the brain (globus pallidus internus and subthalamic nucleus) that control motor movement.

DBS is especially effective for patients who have experienced wearing off of drugs and dyskinesia.

Most post-surgery patients experience benefits of more on time and reduction of involuntary movement. This usually allows them to reduce their dosage of medication. But not all Parkinson's patients are good candidates for DBS, including individuals who are experiencing dementia.

Patients considering this surgical intervention should consult with their doctor about the timing and need for DBS. Normally, deep brain stimulation surgery will be considered when drug treatment is becoming less effective or creating undesirable side effects. There are some risks associated with DBS, including bleeding in the brain and infection.

Research is continuing to discover new medical procedures for the treatment of Parkinson's. One area of promising research is restorative neurosurgery.

This procedure involves the transplanting of dopamine neurons into the brain. Another tantalizing possibility is the transplanting of "stem cells into the brain." Researchers are also examining genetic re-programming of cells in the brain.

These and other procedures currently being researched and developed offer hope for future interventions that can significantly alter or perhaps even cure the ravages of Parkinson's disease.

This is an exciting time in the search for mitigation of symptoms and a cure for Parkinson's disease. Through the efforts of Michael J. Fox, Mohammed Ali, Davis Phinney, and other high profile individuals, attention has been focused on this disease, raising awareness and stimulating funding for research. The Parkinson's community remains hopeful that medical procedures will be identified that may prevent, arrest, and even cure Parkinson's, perhaps in our lifetime.

You Are the Most Important Member of Your Health Care Team

As indicated at the beginning of this chapter, we have intended only to provide a general overview of current medications and other medical interventions for treatment for Parkinson's. Determining the optimum blend of drug interventions for each individual can be frustratingly elusive for you and your doctor. We encourage you to educate yourself on the benefits and potential risks of commonly prescribed medications and therapies—especially those that you are currently taking.

Armed with "basic knowledge," you will be better prepared to partner with your doctor to determine the most effective treatment plan for you.

As emphasized throughout this book, individuals react differently to drugs prescribed for Parkinson's. Your active engagement and feedback can be critical in helping your doctor better understand how you are relating to prescribed drugs—benefits and side effects—and in adjusting your medication plan, as needed. Ultimately, you are the final decision-maker in determining your treatment plan. You are not a passive participant. You have a role, a responsibility to actively participate.

Medications and perhaps even surgical procedures will be the cornerstone of your personal plan for living positively with Parkinson's. But to maximize the benefits of these, you will need to complement them with other physical and emotional health care strategies. Many symptoms of Parkinson's also can be managed with non-drug related therapies and interventions: exercise, physical therapy, occupational therapy, voice therapy, nutrition, and psychological counseling. These and other strategies are covered in other chapters.

As you learn to manage your medications, perhaps no other person will be more intimately involved than your caregiver. From learning together how to pronounce the names of the medications to understanding what each class of medications does, you and your caregiver will be learning a new language together. We will explore the dynamics of caregiving in the next chapter.

NUGGETS

- Developing and managing your medication plan is the most important element of living positively with Parkinson's. Having a basic understanding of drugs prescribed for Parkinson's will enable you to work with your doctor to assess and adjust your medication treatment as you transition through the stages of Parkinson's.

- Some symptoms of Parkinson's also can be managed with surgical and other medical procedures. Deep brain stimulation is currently the most common and effective procedure, but research is continuing to discover new and promising treatments for Parkinson's.

- For the near future, medications will continue to be the primary treatment for Parkinson's, but you may want to talk with your doctor about potential benefits to you of emerging medical interventions.

CHAPTER 6

Caring for the Caregiver

*There are only four kinds of people in this world –
those who have been caregivers, those who are
currently caregivers, those who will be caregivers and
those who will need caregivers.*

—ROSALYN CARTER

"**I** guess I'm a family caregiver," she realized
about six months into their unplanned adventure.

A couple of days later, she informed her husband.

*"You have to be nice to me, you know. I'm your
caregiver!"*

*"You've always been my caregiver," he quipped
back. "I would have been gone a long time ago
without you!"*

They laughed. And in the silence that followed, their smiles acknowledged a deeper truth than their words could explain.

Who is a Caregiver?

According to the Caregiver Action Network, "Caregiving may be one of the most important roles you will ever take on in your life. It is not an easy role, and most of us are never prepared for it. Being a family caregiver for a spouse, parent, child or loved one takes a lot of time, effort and work. It challenges you both intellectually and emotionally. You may have become a caregiver suddenly and without warning, or perhaps your role evolved slowly over time."

According to an older and widely distributed definition, "Family caregiving is the act of assisting someone you care about who is chronically ill or disabled and who is no longer able to care for themselves." Of course, a family caregiver may also be a friend or neighbor. Essentially, if you are taking care of or looking after anyone, you are a caregiver!

Isn't it interesting that we must obtain a license to drive, a degree or certification for our employment, and other certifications for a variety of other endeavors, but nothing at all is required for one of our most likely experiences in life? Moreover, this highly probable scenario of family caregiving will consume an amazing amount of our time and energy.

Did you know that there are about 65 million of us? That's more than one out of every five Americans! About 30% of U.S. households report that at least one person provides care for a chronically ill, disabled or aged family member or friend during any given year and spend an average of 20 hours per week providing care for their loved one. In fact, a 2013 Pew Research release concludes that 39% or "4 out of 10 U.S. adults are caring for a loved one with significant health issues."

Gail Sheehy gives a wonderful description of the caregiver in her book, *Passages in Caregiving*:

"HELP WANTED: Untrained family member or friend to act as advocate, researcher, care manager, and emotional support for a parent or spouse, sibling or friend, who has been diagnosed with a serious illness or chronic disability. Duties: Make medical decisions, negotiate with insurance companies or Medicare; pay bills; legal work; personal care and entertainment in hospital and rehab. Aftercare at home: Substitute for skilled nurse if injections, IV, oxygen, wound care or tube feedings are required. Long-term care: Medication management, showering, toileting, lifting, transporting, etc. Hours: On demand. Salary and benefits: $0."

Family caregivers all deserve a parade, a holiday, and a trip to Disneyworld! If you are a family caregiver, this chapter will provide valuable information for you.

Caregiving 101

As a caregiver, the truth will ultimately be your friend. Granted, reality will deal bitter blows. But, as you acknowledge each change for what it is, you will find that you make better decisions in a timelier manner. You can do this!

In order to manage the demands of being a family caregiver, you will need to keep these suggestions in mind:

- Attend support group meetings

- Exercise regularly

- Make time for friends

- Make necessary changes in the house

- Ask for help when you need it

- Plan for the future

- Don't do everything

- Enjoy the little things

Transitions to Expect

Family caregivers and care receivers experience challenging transitions.

Concerning time perspective, change may burst into your life in an acute manner or it may emerge as a chronic situation that lingers for decades. But, the nuts and bolts of the changes and the difficult dynamics of the transitions test even the most solid people.

First, family caregivers and their loved ones typically face a change in health. With Parkinson's disease, you may notice some symptoms such as stiffness, lack of flexibility, or slight tremors first. If you have lived with even a relatively clean bill of health, these unwelcome physical changes can be highly disorienting.

Often, the ramifications of physical changes include financial implications as more and more of your money is required for medications, doctors, and eventually the need for personal care. Some of the more excruciating changes are related to driving and the home. And of course, helping your family member or friend think about their legacy and prepare to die presents terrain that many of us would rather avoid.

Whether you see these in your immediate future or not, you would be wise to give some consideration to these likely transitions:

- Health

- Driving

- Home

- Finances

- Mental

- Protection

- Legacy and Death

Perhaps these likely scenarios are sending uncomfortable shocks through your system. Do not be overwhelmed.

You can do this! But, you must begin preparing now.

For each transition you are experiencing or can see developing, help is available. Others have walked similar paths before you, and professional resources can assist you in your journey through difficult terrain as well.

As Denise Brown suggests when facing difficult conversations, "Simple is your friend. Think of a simple way to start the conversation."

The three suggestions that follow, if practiced consistently, will place you in a rhythm for living optimally as a family caregiver or as the care receiver.

Care for Caregivers

What refills your cup? A late night or early morning walk? Long baths? Watching movies? Reading? Meditation, prayer, or listening? Bird watching? Golf? Tennis? Exercise? Gardening?

Three suggestions in this section will get you started in the right direction. First of all, **do something for yourself, by yourself, at least weekly if not daily.**

I know what you're thinking; "I don't have time for any of this!" I realize your time is consumed and your energy is low. That is precisely why this suggestion is so crucial. *You must re-energize, re-fill your cup, and re-invigorate your soul.* You cannot afford to skip self-care!

If you have ever flown on an airplane, you know that prior to take-off, the flight attendant emerges from the cabin and gives some counterintuitive instructions. "If we lose cabin pressure, the oxygen masks will fall. After you freak out and scream for a moment (they don't say this, but they might as well), put the oxygen mask on yourself, then help the person next to you."

Why put the mask on yourself first? Simple.

If you are not breathing, you will be of no help to the person next to you.

Translation for family caregivers: If you don't take care of yourself, you will not be able to care for your loved one very well or for very long. Do something for yourself, by yourself, at least weekly.

When we (Bruce) first moved back to Oklahoma City and I led the Caregiver Fundamentals Project, I drove past a cemetery every day on my way home from work. As a hobby, I love to hike, climb, and camp. However, with an ailing wife and two pre-school children, my time was quite limited.

Instead of hiking or camping, I took a walk in the cemetery about once a week. I know, this is not for everyone, especially if you have experienced a recent loss. Yet for at least two reasons, cemeteries provide a great place to refill your cup.

First, no one bothers you. They assume you are either grieving or off your rocker! I assume both applied in my case.

Second, cemeteries can reframe your perspective. After considerable personal research, I can tell you that 90% of those few words we leave behind on a tombstone are about faith and family. The other 10% refers to country.

As I walk around a cemetery, I wonder, "How did these people live? What problems did they experience?" I don't really know. I check dates and realize that some people lived without their spouse for many years. I see that some died too young. But, I don't really know whether they embraced their capacity for resilience or wilted into a lifelong depression.

As I pondered these thoughts week after week, I always came away with the same conclusion. I did not plan on or ask for our circumstances. We did not plan for my wife to get sick or to experience the financial, emotional, and career ramifications that came along with it. But, it was our reality.

Then, the sun would rise again in my mind as I thought, "I still have my wife. My children still have their mommy. It's not ideal, but it's what we have.

For that, I am thankful. I'm going home now to make the best of it."

I love this suggestion and language from Gail Sheehy: "Reconnect with your transports to joy." Beautiful. But, how do you do it and what does this mean?

Reconnect with your transports to joy?

What fills your cup? Long walks, music, art, reading, cooking, or creating help many people. In order for you to reconnect with your transports to joy, you must ruthlessly carve out a sacred space and time to engage in these life-giving moments.

Yes, I realize that time may be hard to find. But, if you are going to live well through this situation, you must allow yourself space. Remember, you have permission to care for yourself.

The second suggestion in this section is to connect with people who fill your cup at least weekly.

Some people fill your cup; some people drain your cup.

Stay away from the later, and seek out the former!

If you have a support group, small group, dinner group, or breakfast group that rejuvenates you, intentionally create time to make those gatherings happen. If you know an individual you can talk to on the phone or meet with regularly who lifts your spirits, etch those encouragement sessions into your schedule.

For me, the answer was a weekly breakfast with friends at the Classen Grill. Each Thursday morning around 7:00 a.m., I met three or four friends at this iconic establishment. The energy in this greasy spoon surged with life. A favorite meeting spot for state lawmakers and local celebrities, I dined with a sense of adventure. For less than $10 a week, I could sightsee in another universe and enjoy the atmosphere, Chinook eggs, good friends, and a waitress who called me "hun."

Like me, my friends were working their way up various career ladders. All in our early thirties at the time, opportunities arose regularly. Most of our conversation revolved around our new forays and discoveries.

We talked very little about our struggles. Most of them had no experience or vocabulary to offer me. Their wives had not been sick. Most of their lives resonated with a much more carefree tone than mine.

And that was okay. I needed their friendship, their half-true stories, and the excitement of being young. I am so thankful for those friends during that painful time. Even now, I resist tears as I remember.

Who are your people? Perhaps you are thinking of long-time friends, church friends, or fellow travelers in a support group. Maybe your breakfast group, coffee group, or exercise buddies come to mind. But, find the people who fill your cup and connect with them. Then, stay connected.

Maybe you need people who can listen and give you wise counsel. But, perhaps you just need to get away and *not think about it.* Whether you are the caregiver or the patient, you need to connect to the people who fill your cup.

During the same years I was having breakfast each week at Classen Grill, my wife was enjoying the friendship of the ladies in our small group from church. Their sorority gelled quickly as a mutually supportive gathering of encouragement and open sharing.

Words truly fall short as I recall how important those relationships have been for my wife. Her friends supplied what I could not. And again, I am thankful.

When the Parkinson Foundation of Oklahoma introduced voice therapy groups, we expected the therapy to help people speak louder. But after a few months, we noticed that people kept returning for another reason. They relished the friendships and sense of newfound community with people who shared their path.

Find *your* people. Get and stay connected.

The third and final suggestion is to ask for help.

For those of us who prefer to give help, asking for help poses a major challenge.

The truth is that most of us do need help at some point.

Or, things would at least go much more smoothly if we would simply ask.

Asking for assistance does *not* mean that you are helpless. It *does* mean that you are humble and smart. You put your pride on hold for a greater good, and you are keen enough to do the right thing.

At some point along the way, you may need counseling, financial advice or assistance, more disease information, meals, or help cleaning the house. You may find that in-home care, home health, hospice, assisted living, or care coordination would be helpful.

When my wife was still in the first year of her illness, I was working as a minister at a church. One day, a distraught lady came to me for counsel. Her daughter had been diagnosed with a severe illness and her mother was quite literally lying on her deathbed.

She was experiencing depression. I could easily see and diagnose the symptoms, so I offered her encouragement and helped arrange sessions with someone better trained than I.

As she left my office, I closed the door and leaned back against it. My head dropped. "She's not the only one who is depressed," I spoke softly to myself. "So am I."

I have always assumed that it is good for other people to visit with a counselor or therapist. In fact, I have helped many people arrange or finance their sessions.

This time, I discovered that it was a good idea for me as well. The sessions I invested in counseling were just what I needed: someone to help me sort things out and navigate my way out of a season of depression.

Help has come in numerous forms on our journey. From meals to counseling to assistance from my in-laws and my parents, we have needed extra hands and feet as we have dealt with my wife's illness.

Tell the truth.

What help do you need to ask for right now?

If you are not sure what steps to take next, please visit the "Recommended Resources" and appendix for leads.

Additionally, you might consider these 10 Tips for Family Caregivers from the National Family Caregiver Association:

1. Seek support from other caregivers. You are not alone!

2. Take care of your own health so that you can be strong enough to take care of your loved one.

3. Accept offers of help and suggest specific things people can do to help you.

4. Learn how to communicate effectively with doctors.

5. Caregiving is hard work so take respite breaks often.

6. Watch out for signs of depression and don't delay in getting professional help when you need it.

7. Be open to new technologies that can help you care for your loved one.

8. Organize medical information so it's up to date and easy to find.

9. Make sure legal documents are in order.

10. Give yourself credit for doing the best you can in one of the toughest jobs there is!

From the shock of initial diagnosis to partnering with others to build a team around you, you are learning to cope and to live well with Parkinson's. You can do this!

Join us in chapter seven for a jolt of practical guidance and encouragement. Take courage!

NUGGETS

- Having a caregiver is crucial to maintaining a meaningful quality of life for people with Parkinson's, especially in the disease's advanced stages. A caregiver is usually a family member but can also be a close relative or trusted friend. It is estimated that 65 million, one in every five people, in America are caregivers.

- If you are a caregiver you will experience challenging transitions and increasing demands on your physical and emotional resources as your loved one's disease progresses. Self-care is essential for caregivers. Simply stated, if you don't take care of yourself, you will not be able to care for your loved one very well or very long.

- Don't try to carry your burden alone; seek help when you need it. Develop an informal group of friends who "fill your cup," and take time away from your caregiving duties to spend time with them, weekly or as needed. You also may want to seek help from a mental health professional. In the late stages of your caregiving, you may find that in-home care, assisted living, or care coordination will be helpful or even necessary.

CHAPTER 7

Living Positively With Parkinson's

When there is no hope in the future there is no power in the present.
—JOHN MAXWELL

Near the end of their first year with Parkinson's, John and Mary got away to a cabin for a week. Sitting on the deck overlooking a bend in the river, they sipped their morning coffee.

"You know, it's been about a year," John offered.

"Yes, and I think we've come a long way," Mary said with a bit of hope.

"I think we're doing the right things to live well with PD," John observed. *"Not that everything's perfect, but we're doing what we know to do and it's helping."*

"I agree and I'm proud of you," Mary said with an old admiration in her eyes.

With a sense of gratitude for where they were on the journey thus far, they smiled, sipped their coffee, and enjoyed the moment.

Your Holistic Plan

Having journeyed with us this far, we assume that you have owned your Parkinson's disease.

You have resolved to be proactive not passive, hopeful not helpless.

You have educated yourself on this complex and sometimes baffling disease called Parkinson's, dispelling myths and misinformation. You have acquired important basic knowledge about the physical, mental, and emotional disabilities of this disease. And, you understand medications, medical procedures, and other health care interventions for treating and living successfully with Parkinson's. Hopefully, this information has motivated you to prepare a personalized, evolving wellness plan. This plan will help you integrate these available resources and provide you with a roadmap for implementing your health care strategies.

Now, we encourage you to take an additional courageous, bold, and potentially life-altering step on your journey with Parkinson's.

Think deeply about emotional, spiritual, and other personal assets you can invest in your Parkinson's plan.

This is more than just positive thinking, though an attitude of positive expectancy is necessary. We are asking you to transform your basic Parkinson's plan into a "holistic plan" that includes these additional resources.

Parkinson's changes you forever. It will require you to consider choices and make fundamental changes in your life to accommodate its progressively debilitating physical and emotional outcomes. Perhaps for the first time, you will consider your own human frailty. Will you be a victim or victor? Proactive or passive? The title of this book suggests its central themes of hope and "strength for the journey" that empower you to live positively and victoriously with Parkinson's.

Dr. Michael S. Okun is the National Medical Director for the National Parkinson Foundation, a prolific researcher, and an internationally recognized authority on Parkinson's disease treatment. Dr.

Okun emphasizes in his book, *Parkinson's Treatment: 10 Secrets to A Happier Life* that,

"The journey of the Parkinson's disease patient is fueled by hope.

I have come to realize that it is the hope that ultimately leads to their happiness." And he concludes that, "It is the hope that will continue to define them through the sometimes difficult journey."

Cram, Schechter, and Gao in their book, *Understanding Parkinson's Disease: A Self-Help Guide,* emphasize that, "Our minds and bodies are connected," and "your attitude is perhaps the most essential element of self-help." And in concluding remarks, they affirm that, "we must never give up hope....The joy in life comes from inside each of us." The authors of *Parkinson Positive* share this philosophy and the importance of a positive and proactive role of the patient in managing Parkinson's disease.

The "Positives" in Your Life

As a first step in developing your enhanced, holistic plan, consider this.

Compile a comprehensive list of all the positives in your life.

Refer to this list frequently. It could include a hundred items and even more. And it likely might include: a loving spouse, caring family members, supportive friends, a strong religious faith, a home, personal freedoms, special skills, financial resources, dedicated health care providers, hobbies and creative interests, emotional reserves, and personal goals that you still can achieve. The list could and should continue. Researcher and author on positive psychology, Christopher Peterson, adds, "Good days have common features: feeling autonomous, competent, and connected to others."

Focusing on these positives will provide you a more realistic and balanced perspective for your life and help you develop what Zig Ziglar referred to as an "attitude of gratitude."

The key is to focus on what you have and can do, not what you don't have and can't do.

Remind yourself regularly of the gifts and graces you have been given. Reflect on the good people and good things in your life, especially on those down days when you are assailed by doubt and fear. American entrepreneur Henry Ford pointed out that, "Whether you think you can, or think you can't... you are right." Think you can and believe you can live positively with Parkinson's!

The Precious Present

An unexpected positive outcome of having Parkinson's is the opportunity to think seriously about important matters.

Reassess your values, priorities, and life goals in light of your disabilities.

Knowing how many quality years of life (hopefully several) you have remaining can give you a sense of urgency to act and do while you can. But it also calls you to reflect on and make time for people and activities that are of high value to you. Spencer Johnson, in his book, *The Precious Present,* teaches us that we can learn to experience and cherish each day, each moment as it comes to us: "My past was the present. And my future will be the present. The present moment is the only reality I ever experience." Learn to live in the moment.

Charles Hummel in his classic and timeless booklet, *Tyranny of the Urgent,* reminds us that, "The urgent task calls for instant action....But in the light of time's perspective, their deceptive prominence fades; with a sense of loss we recall the vital task we pushed aside. We realize we've become slaves to the tyranny of the urgent." With the precious remaining time you (and all of us) have, don't let the urgent things crowd out the important things in your life.

Choose how and with whom you will want to share the precious present.

Declining physical energy and mental acumen likely will impact your ability to handle multiple priorities like you have in the past. As you reassess your priorities, are there activities and commitments that you can say "no" to, allowing you to say "yes" to more important priorities?

Are there important things that you have put off and words of love and forgiveness left unspoken? Have you sacrificed quality time with your spouse, family members, and special friends for urgent things? Are there hobbies and special interests that you intend to pursue some day and bucket list items that you have always planned to do but "just haven't gotten around to?" Don't waste this life-changing opportunity to reassess your activities and commitments and realign them with your revised priorities.

Sustaining Energy

Living positively with Parkinson's will, to a large degree, depend on your ability to achieve and sustain physical and emotional energy on a daily basis.

Legendary football coach Vince Lombardi observed that, "Fatigue makes cowards of us all." When we are physically and emotionally fatigued, we often give in and give up. This is especially true for people with Parkinson's, who struggle with serious health issues. It is so tempting, when you are tired, to stoop and shuffle your feet when walking, to not stretch and exercise regularly, to not work on your voice exercises, to be negative and irritable, to withdraw from social activities, and to just generally feel sorry for yourself.

Undergirding your holistic plan for living positively with Parkinson's is the amount of energy that you can consistently bring to each day and to each moment. As Coach Lombardi pointed out,

Fatigue is our enemy.

We have discussed the importance of proper dosage and timing of medication, diet, exercise, and sleep in maintaining physical energy. And it is equally critical to include in your wellness plan a regimen of activities to help you sustain your emotional reserves.

Prominent Harvard psychologist Will James explained that,

"We can change our lives by altering our attitudes."

Writing and reciting positive affirmations is a powerful tool for maintaining a positive attitude. These can be personal statements you write up or inspirational quotes that speak to you. Post them around your home and place them in your purse or wallet. Read or recite them to yourself when experiencing doubt, when feeling tired, before important activities or events, before exercising or taking medications, and any time negative thoughts or feelings of inadequacy and despair assail you.

Feed your brain positive food.

Weave relaxing moments into your daily life. Read and listen to inspirational literature and tapes, listen to relaxing music, refer to your list of positives, laugh often, and love unconditionally. Spend quality time with family, and reconnect with old friends. Participate in activities of service to others, and set aside time to engage in hobbies and special interests that give you satisfaction and a sense of self-worth. Possibilities for positive renewal are endless. Living Parkinson's positive is an act of will. Napoleon Hill and W. Clement Stone in their book, *Success Through A Positive Mental Attitude*, affirmed that, "What the mind can conceive and believe—the mind can achieve."

Renowned psychologist Martin Seligman emphasizes five research-based elements of well-being. These include positive emotion, engagement, meaning, accomplishment, and positive relationships. To gauge your attunement to these elements, you might consider the following questions:

- Do you intentionally create pleasant experiences throughout your day?

- Do you engage in a hobby or project in which you become completely absorbed and perhaps lose track of time?

- Do you belong to or serve in some way that you believe is bigger than yourself?

- Are you in the habit of regularly achieving, completing, or accomplishing goals or even small tasks?

- Finally, are you consistently laughing, talking, and spending time with other people?

If the rhythm of your life moves to these beats, you are likely to experience well-being.

Spiritual Resources

For many Parkinson's patients, the cornerstone of their plan to combat Parkinson's is the sustaining power of spirituality. Christians, Jews, Muslims, Hindus, Buddhists, and other religious believers have access to a greater power beyond themselves that can comfort, sustain, and empower them. The power of prayer and faith when combined with medical interventions can provide positive and sometimes even miraculous outcomes.

Your religious faith can sustain you and provide hope and assurance.

It provides peace, joy, hope, and emotional strength for the journey, wherever it takes you and however it ends.

Journey's End

It is a truism that, "we are all born terminal; we just don't know the date." When their symptoms are appropriately managed, most people with Parkinson's will live, on average, only two or three years less than a comparable pool of individuals without the disease. But due to the disease's potentially life-altering disabilities, such as dementia, it is important to be ready.

Prepare in advance for possible incapacitating outcomes and end of life issues.

Parkinson's patients should consider writing legal directives that spell out how they want their legal, financial, and health care issues to be handled should they become emotionally or mentally incapable of managing their personal affairs. These directives will usually include: an authorized signer on their bank account, durable power of attorney, living trust, health care directive, advance directive ("living will"), and other documents as needed.

Information on these financial and legal directives is included in the appendix of this book, under the title, "Preparation For Incapacitating and End of Life Events." A thorough and detailed discussion of financial and legal issues is included in Parashos, Wichmann, and Melby, *Navigating Life with Parkinson Disease.*

It is important that you include your spouse, if still living, in this planning process and that you meet with your family and other appropriate individuals to share and discuss your legal documents and health care directives. Allow them to ask questions, offer suggestions, and understand your intentions. Based on these candid conversations, you may want to make some revisions. Keep at least one copy of your legal instruments in a secure place outside your home and share copies, as needed, with family members. Periodically review your documents, directives, and other instructions, and revise them when necessary.

You might want to discuss and share with your family, in writing, how you want your celebration of life service and burial or cremation details to be handled. Give them a list of individuals (include contact information) to be notified. And provide them with information for inclusion in newspaper notices and obituaries. Don't leave difficult decisions about providing for you should you become incapacitated or when you decease to your spouse and children in these emotionally stressful times.

Providing instructions for end of life contingencies can be your final gift of love to those you love.

Circle of Life

The circle is closed. We begin and end with the overarching themes of hope and proactive self-management.

You are in control and despite debilitating disabilities you can live Parkinson positive.

We reaffirm that it is absolutely critical that first you develop a medical intervention plan. It should include appropriate medication, necessary therapies, diet, and exercise, and a team of physicians and skilled health care providers to help you implement your personal plan. But we also have asked you to consider untapped mental, emotional, and spiritual reserves that you can invest in your holistic plan. These intangible resources can provide emotional strength for the journey, keep you focused on your plan, and help you live positively with Parkinson's.

NUGGETS

- The foundation of your plan to live successfully with Parkinson's is appropriate medication, necessary therapies, mental health care, diet, and exercise. But, to live Parkinson positive you will need to invest your mental, emotional, and spiritual resources in an enhanced holistic plan.

- An unexpected positive outcome of having Parkinson's is the opportunity to reassess your values, priorities, and life goals in light of your disabilities. You may find that urgent things have crowded out more important things in your life. Don't waste this opportunity to reassess your activities and commitments and realign them with your revised priorities

- Due to Parkinson's potentially life-altering outcomes, including dementia, it is especially important to prepare early for possible incapacitating outcomes and end of life issues. You should consider legal documents that spell out how you want your estate to be handled and your assets to be distributed when you decease. You also should write legal directives that spell out how you want your legal, financial, and health care issues to be handled should you become emotionally or mentally incapacitated.

Conclusion

Our journey together through the pages of this book has ended. Along the way you have acquired knowledge and a positive perspective on living with Parkinson's that will provide hope and strength for your continuing journey.

Another purpose of this book is to provide you with a medical tool box to keep in arm's reach and consult frequently. "Take Action" guidelines and other practical tools included in the appendix will help you build and update your evolving Parkinson's plan. And when you seek authoritative information beyond the scope of this book, we encourage you to refer to the "Recommended Resources."

We leave you with this self-actualizing truth. You are not defined by your disease. Davis Phinney, a national spokesperson for living victoriously with Parkinson's, emphasizes that,

"You can't control that you have Parkinson's, but you can control what you do about it."

And Michael J. Fox reminds us, "I have no choice about whether or not I have Parkinson's; I have nothing but choices about how I react to it."

And in your choices lies your hope.

Choose well. Your authors wish you Godspeed on your continuing journey and pray that you choose always to be Parkinson positive.

Take Action

- Date you were diagnosed:

- What you need to learn next:

- Things I **can't** control:

- Things I **can** control:

- Name of your neurologist. If you don't have a neurologist, ask for a referral or call a Parkinson's organization near you for recommendations.

- Members of your healthcare team:
  Neurologist:
  General Physician:
  Physical Therapist:
  Voice Therapist:
  Nutritionist:

Counselor:

- What three things can you do to help your family and friends help you?

- What symptoms are affecting your activities of daily living and how are you coping?

- New coping techniques to experiment with:

- What questions do you need to ask your neurologist? Is it about your medications or daily coping rhythms?

- How are you or your caregiver:

- ○ Doing something for yourself by yourself to refill your cup weekly if not daily?

- ○ Connecting with people who fill your cup?

- ○ Asking for help?

- What further actions do you need to take to live *Parkinson's positive*?

Endnotes

Chapter One

4 *Up to 1.5 million* "Moving Forward: A Practical Guide to Living with Parkinson's Disease, 3rd Edition," *Teva Neuroscience* (2010): 15.

4 *double to 30 million world-wide* Michael S. Okun, *Parkinson's Treatment: 10 Secrets to a Happier Life* (Amazon, 2013), vii, xi.

5 *parkinsonisms* J. Eric Ahlskog, *The Parkinson's Disease Treatment Book: Partnering with Your Doctor to Get the Most from Your Medications* (Oxford University Press, 2005), 57-82.

Dr. Ahlskog presents with scientific thoroughness the difficult process of discerning Parkinson's from other diseases with similar symptoms. And he emphasizes the importance of confirming a Parkinson's diagnosis early to initiate appropriate medical intervention.

5 *neurologist specializing in movement disorders*

See additional information on selecting a neurologist in chapter two.

8   *die 'with' rather than die 'from'*   Sotirios A. Parashos, Rose Wichmann, and Todd Melby, *Navigating Life with Parkinson's Disease* (Oxford University Press, 2005), 30.

8   *How many years of life do I have remaining?*

An informative study on longevity of Parkinson's patients   conducted by Mayo Clinic is referenced in Ahlskog, *The Parkinson's Disease Treatment Book*, 49.

11   *genes load the gun*   Okun, *Parkinson's Treatment*, 80.

14   *wide array of...debilitating disabilities*

These symptoms and disabilities are listed later in this chapter. For more in-depth information identifying and describing these, refer to the following books, which both devote two chapters to this topic: Ahlskog, *The Parkinson's Disease Treatment Book*, 25-74, and

Parashos, Wichmann, Melby, *Navigating Life with Parkinson's Disease*, 33-70.

Chapter Two

21 *Reducing your PD symptoms*

The Parkinson Foundation of Oklahoma has found a great partner in TEVA Neuroscience. Their publication, *Moving Forward*, p. 19, provided insight into personal priorities for developing a game plan that we found difficult to improve upon.

22 *Partner—that was the word we were looking for* Gail Sheehy, *Passages in Caregiving*: *Turning Chaos into Confidence* (New York: HarperCollins Publishers, 2010), 19.

23 *The more educated and experienced a person becomes in their field* Malcolm Gladwell, *Blink* (New York: Little, Brown and Company, 2005), 3-16.

While this book is not specifically about PD or neurology, the author makes an overwhelming case for the advantages of the expert eye on any given situation.

23 *consider these additional questions*

AGIS.com (Assist Guide Information Services)

This website provides plentiful resources including checklists for almost any care situation or transition.

27 *Regular exercise benefits people with Parkinson's disease*

http://pdcenter.neurology.ucsf.edu/patients-guide (Parkinson's Disease Clinic and Research Center)

28 *89% of Parkinson patients* Lorraine Ramig, et al. "Speech treatment for Parkinson's disease," *Expert Review of Neurotherapeutics Journal* (February 2008): 299-311.

28 *It is possible to save a voice*

Samantha Elandary, founder and CEO of the Parkinson Voice Project. Go to parkinsonvoiceproject.org/kasem.html to learn more about their effective therapy.

29   *Occupational Therapy (OT) may be able to help*

http://www.pdf.org/en/science_news/release/pr_1400 260722 (Parkinson Disease Foundation, posted May 16, 2014)

30   *about 50% of patients with PD experience depression* Irene Richard and Roger Kurlan, "The under-recognition of depression in Parkinson's disease," *Neuropsychiatric Disease and Treatment* (September 2006): 349-353.

Chapter Three

34   *Vulnerability isn't good or bad* Brene Brown, *Daring Greatly* (New York: Penguin Group, 2012), 33.

37   *Consider your experiences thus far from the template of: Challenge, choices, outcomes*

This helpful model comes from Bill Moyer's program "How to tell your story of self" with credit given to 350.org workshops. To learn more, visit http://workshops.350.org/toolkit/story/.

Chapter Four

48 *Most people with Parkinson's experience dysphagia*

http://www.epda.eu.com/en/x-parkinsons/in-depth/pdsymptoms/eating-swallowing/ (European Parkinson Disease Association)

49 *schedule meals during "on" time* National Parkinson Foundation, *Activities of Daily Living: Practical Pointers for Parkinson's Disease*, 22.

You can find this publication at http://www3.parkinson.org/site/DocServer/Practical_P ointers.pdf?docID=194.

50 *According to the Aged Carer*

http://www.agedcarer.com.au/topic/aged-care-health-issues/parkinsons-disease-and-everyday-tips#hygiene

51 *Rigid muscles, tremor*

http://www.pdf.org/en/sleep_disturbance
(Parkinson Disease Foundation on "Sleep Disturbances")

52   *keep a regular sleep schedule*

http://sleepfoundation.org/sleep-topics/parkinsons-disease-and-sleep/page/0/3
(Sleep Foundation article on Parkinson's disease and sleep)

53   *gait hypokinesia is a characteristic feature*
M.E. Morris, et al., "Ability to modulate walking cadence remains intact in Parkinson's disease," *Journal of Neurology, Neurosurgery, and Psychiatry* v. 57 (December 1994): 1532-1534.

53   *that this therapy is viable in PD* Mirleman, et al. "Virtual reality for gait training: can it enduce motor learning to enhance complex walking and reduce fall risk in patients with Parkinson's disease?" *Journals of Gerontology. Series A, Biological Sciences and Medical Sciences 66, no. 2* (February 2011): 234-240.

54   *Exercise may promote brain repair* M.A. Hirsch and B.G.Farley, "Exercise and neuroplasticity in

persons living with Parkinson's disease," *European Journal of Physical and Rehabilitation Medicine* 45, (2009): 215-229.

56 *Coping...is crucial* Leslie D. Frazier, "Coping with disease-related stressors in Parkinson's disease," *The Gerontologist* 40, no. 1, 53-63.

Chapter Five

Authors' note: multiple primary and secondary sources were consulted to determine content and ensure accuracy of information provided in chapter five. Though sometimes not cited, the following sources helped inform the authors' understanding and presentation of the symptoms and current medical treatments for Parkinson's disease. These specific resources are also listed because they are written for and readily understandably by the lay public. Complete citations with annotations are listed under "Recommended Resources."

J. Eric Ahlskog, *The Parkinson's Disease Treatment Book: Partnering with Your Doctor to Get the Most from Your Medications.*

David L. Cram, Steven H. Schechter, and Xiao-Ke Gao, *Understanding Parkinson's Disease: A Self-*

Help Guide, Second Edition.

Michael Okun, *Parkinson's Treatment: The 10 Secrets to a Happier Life.*

Sotirios A. Parashos, Rose Wichmann, and Todd Melby, *Navigating Life with Parkinson's Disease.*

69 *timing of medication dosages* Okun, *Parkinson's Treatment, 20.*

73 *Deep brain stimulation (DBS)*

Parashos, Wichmann, and Melby, *Navigating Life with Parkinson Disease*, pp. 130-141; Okun, *Parkinson's Treatment*, pp. 23-30; and J. Eric Ahlskog, *The Parkinson's Disease Treatment Book*, pp. 473-486, discuss this surgical procedure in detail, including potential benefits and risks and information about patients who may not be good candidates for DBS.

Chapter Six

79 *caregiving may be one of the most*

http://www.caregiveraction.org/resources/
(Caregiver Action Network)

Additionally, the following quote comes from earlier literature and websites by their former name, the National Family Caregiver Association.

80   *4 out of 10 U.S. adults* Drew DeSilver, "As population ages, more Americans become caregivers," Pew Research Center, July 18, 2013, http://www.pewresearch.org/fact-tank/2013/07/18/as-population-ages-more-americans-becoming-caregivers/.

80   *Help Wanted* Sheehy, *Passages in Caregiving,* 10.

81   *Attend support group meetings* Parashos, *Navigating Life*, 224-25.

82-90

Much of the content in these pages is adapted from *Graceful Transitions*, one of Bruce McIntyre's previous works.

84   *simple is your friend* Denise Brown, *The Caregiving Years, Six Stages to a Meaningful*

Journey (Chicago: Tad Publishing, 2013), 14.

87 *reconnect with your transports to joy* Sheehy, *Passages in Caregiving,* 261.

92 *seek support from other caregivers*

http://www.caregiveraction.org/resources/ten-tips (Caregiver Action Network)

Chapter Seven

98 *The journey of the Parkinson's patient* Okun, *Parkinson's Treatment,* p. 95; David L. Cram, Steven H. Schechter, and Xiao-Ke Gao, *Understanding Parkinson's Disease* (Omaha: Addicus Books, 2009), 1-2, 123.

99 *good days have common features* Christopher Peterson, *Pursuing the Good Life* (New York: Oxford University Press, 2013), 5.

100 *we can learn to experience and cherish each day* Spencer Johnson, *The Precious Present* (Garden City, New York: Doubleday & Company, 1984), 67.

100 *The urgent task calls for instance action*
Charles Hummel, *Tyranny of the Urgent* (Downers
Grove, IL: InterVarsity Christian Fellowship of the
United States of America, 1967), 9-10.

Hummel is also quoted in: Stephen R. Covey, A.
Roger Merrill, and Rebecca R. Merrill, *First Things
First: To Live, to Love, to Leave A Legacy* (New York:
A Fireside Book, Simon & Schuster, 1994), 36.

103 *Living Parkinson's positive is an act of will*
Napoleon Hill and W. Clement Stone, *Success
Through A Positive Mental Attitude* (Englewood
Cliffs, New Jersey: Prentice Hall, 1960), 25.

104 *five research-based elements of well-being*
Martin Seligman, *Flourish* (New York: Free Press,
2011), 16-21.

Seligman is one of the fathers of the new era of
positive psychology, which emphasizes a holistic
notion of well-being.

106 *A thorough and detailed discussion of financial
and legal issues* Murray Sagsveen and Laurie
Hanson, "Planning for Your Future: Managing Your

Personal Affairs," chapter 13, in Parashos, Wichmann, and Melby, *Navigating Life with Parkinson's Disease*, pp. 235-259.

This chapter includes an informative and comprehensive discussion of legal, financial, and health care directives for Parkinson's patients and their families to consider in preparation for possible incapacitating events and end of life issues.

Recommended Resources

BOOKS

Ahlskog, J. Eric. *The Parkinson's Disease Treatment Book: Partnering with Your Doctor to Get the Most from Your Medications.* New York: Oxford University Press, 2005. Dr. Ahlskog is Chair of the Mayo Section of Movement Disorders, Mayo Clinic, and a leading authority on Parkinson's disease. This comprehensive guide is especially noteworthy for its scholarly and yet readable information on medications and other medical interventions for treatment of Parkinson. A must read for individuals seeking in-depth information on nearly every topic related to Parkinson's.

Ali, Rasheeda. *I'll Hold Your Hand So You Won't Fall.* West Palm Beach: Merit Publishing, 2010. If you are attempting to explain Parkinson's to a child or grandchild, this book may give you some ideas and eliminate unnecessary fear.

Cram, David L., Schechter, Steven H., and Gao, Xiao-Ke. *Understanding Parkinson's Disease: A Self-Help Guide*, Second Edition. Omaha, Nebraska: Addicus Books, 2009. This book emphasizes the crucial role of the patient in managing Parkinson's. Dr. Cram has lived with Parkinson's for twenty-five years, and his personal experiences influence the patient-centric "self-help" theme of the book. The book successfully melds medical treatment and self-treatment into a holistic strategy for achieving quality of life.

McIntyre, Bruce. *Graceful Transitions: An Inspirational Guide for Caregivers and Care Receivers.* Edmond, OK: Rabbit Ranch Press, 2012. In this book, the caregiver will find questions, models, and suggestions that resonate with the daily dynamics of unwelcome change in the care situation.

Okun, Michael S. *Parkinson's Treatment: 10 Secrets to a Happier Life.* Published on Amazon, 2013. Dr. Okun, an authority on Parkinson's treatment and National Medical Director of the National Parkinson Foundation, weaves engaging and compassionate stories of his patient experiences with authoritative information on Parkinson's and its treatment. In addition to providing cutting-edge information, his inspirational book offers hope and "secrets" for living with Parkinson's. Read and re-read this book for those times when you need hope and emotional support.

Parashos, Sotirios A., Wichmann, Rose, and Melby, Todd. *Navigating Life with Parkinson Disease.* New York: Oxford University Press, 2013. This scholarly and comprehensive book is a volume in the American Academy of Neurology's Neurology Now™ book series. The book balances its overarching theme that, "knowledge is empowering," with practical applications for living successfully with Parkinson's.

Sheehy, Gail. *Passages in Caregiving: Turning Chaos Into Confidence.* New York: HarperCollins Publishers, 2010. This volume delivers perhaps the most comprehensive yet readable book on family caregiving to date. With warm narrative and practical advice, the reader will find this book especially helpful through the seasons of care.

WEBSITES

The websites listed below are excellent sources of current information on Parkinson's for patients and their families. Format and content of sites vary, but collectively they include: insightful articles, newsletters, reports on recent research, FAQs, fact sheets, blogs, video clips, online seminars, and live streaming of educational presentations.

As you research online, you will discover other informative and insightful websites in addition to those mentioned here.

ADVOCACY ORGANIZATIONS

American Parkinson's Disease Association
www.apdaparkinson.org.

APDA resources are focused on "research, patient services, education, and raising public awareness for Parkinson's disease." In addition to the comprehensive resources and programs it offers, APDA is a major funder of research on Parkinson's disease.

Davis Phinney Foundation for Parkinson's
www.davisphinneyfoundation.org

This foundation supports research initiatives, sponsors programs, and provides information that focus on helping patients "live well with Parkinson's." The one-day *Victory Summit®* series of symposia offered across the United States is a signature program of the foundation.

Michael J. Fox Foundation for Parkinson's Research
www.michaeljfox.org

This is an information rich website on all aspects of Parkinson's disease, with emphasis on providing support for research to "eliminate Parkinson's disease in our lifetime." It is currently the largest nonprofit funder of Parkinson's research nationally. With helpful videos, guides, and tools, the Michael J. Fox Foundation makes it easy to engage in research and education.

National Parkinson Foundation
www.Parkinson.org

NPF's website provides an extensive array of helpful information, programs, and practical tools for patients, caregivers, and professionals.

Parkinson's Action Network
www.parkinsonsaction.org

PAN is a grassroots advocacy network that seeks to "educate the public and government leaders on better policies for research and improved quality of life for people living with Parkinson's."

Parkinson Alliance
www.parkinsonalliance.org

A major goal of the Parkinson Alliance is raising funds to help finance research on Parkinson's disease.

PD Index—Directory of PD Information on the Internet
www.pdindex.org

The Directory includes an extensive listing of websites related to all aspects of Parkinson's disease.

Parkinson's Disease Foundation
www.pdf.org

The PDF website offers many educational resources (videos, conferences, materials, and information on current research) for patients and professionals.

Parkinson Foundation of Oklahoma
www.parkinsonoklahoma.com

PFO is a nonprofit organization committed to improving the quality of life for Parkinson's patients, families, and caregivers in the State of Oklahoma. Services and programs include: patient and family consultations, "Parkinson's 101" classes, SPEAK OUT® Oklahoma voice enhancement program, and educational conferences for patients and caregivers. PFO also provides resources for Parkinson's support groups and exercise groups across Oklahoma.

WebMD
www.webmd.com

WebMD website offers information on numerous health-related issues, including Parkinson's disease.

CAREGIVING

Assist Guide Information Services
www.agis.com

Assist Guide Information Services has created perhaps the single best website for family caregivers. Be sure to click on the "checklists" button on the left side bar for practical questions to ask about numerous care transitions.

Caregiver.com
www.caregiver.com

Gary Barg leads this extensive site with tons of helpful articles, as well as *Today's Caregiver* magazine.

Caregiver Action Network
www.caregiveraction.org
Formerly known as The National Family Caregiving Association now operates by this name and website.

Caregiving.com
www.caregiving.com
Denise Brown leads this interactive website that delivers solid encouragement and guidance. Incidentally, Bruce McIntyre cohosts a podcast with Denise Brown on this site at the time of this publication.

The Family Caregiver Alliance
www.caregiver.org
The Family Caregiver Alliance pioneered important programs for information, education, services, research, and advocacy and continues to provide reliable help.

The National Alliance for Caregiving
www.caregiving.org
The National Alliance for Caregiving focuses on research and advocacy.

MEDICAL SOCIETIES

American Academy of Neurology
www.AAN.com

This website includes information and educational resources primarily for academy members and other health care professionals.

AAN also manages a website for the lay public (www.thebrainmatters.org). Other resources offered to lay people include the *Neurology Now* magazine and the Neurology Now™ book series for patients and caregivers.

ADDITIONAL RESOURCES

There are numerous insightful and informative books, articles and websites in addition to those mentioned above. The reader is encouraged to refer to sources cited in the text and endnotes of our *Parkinson Positive* book. Bibliographies listed in books included in our "Recommended Resources" are also excellent sources of additional information.

Appendix

WORKSHEETS AND CHECKLISTS

SELECTING A PHYSICIAN

Question	Yes	No	Comments
Is the doctor in your loved one's insurance company's network of providers?			
If not, can you or your loved one afford to cover the costs not covered by the insurance company?			
Is the doctor board certified for the specialty needed?			
Is the doctor affiliated with the preferred hospital?			
Does the doctor take an active interest in your or your caree's health?			
Do you think this doctor will collaborate?			

DOCTOR'S OFFICE VISIT RECORD

Doctor's Name:

Date of Visit:

Reason for Visit:

Symptoms or Concerns: List any new symptoms, pains, or feelings since the last visit. List anything brought up by another physician or health provider.

1.

2.

3.

Questions for the Doctor:

1.

2.

3.

Diagnosis and Course of Treatment:

Special Instructions:

Referral to Another Physician:

MEDICATION LIST

Name: Date of Birth:
Pharmacy Name:
Pharmacy Phone #:
Pharmacy Address:

Drug name:				
Reason for Use				
Prescribing Physician				
Description				
Expiration Date				
Dosage and Frequency				
Special Instructions				
Timing				

CAREGIVER SELF-ASSESSMENT

How often have I lately...	Please rate 1=Never 3=Sometimes 5= Always				
Had trouble staying focused on what I was doing?	1	2	3	4	5
Had difficulty making decisions?	1	2	3	4	5
Felt that I can't leave my caree alone?	1	2	3	4	5
Felt overwhelmed?	1	2	3	4	5
Felt resentful?	1	2	3	4	5
Felt helpless?	1	2	3	4	5
Felt lonely?	1	2	3	4	5
Felt weary or tired?	1	2	3	4	5
Felt anxious?	1	2	3	4	5
Been physically exhausted?	1	2	3	4	5
Been irritable?	1	2	3	4	5
Lost or had poor sleep?	1	2	3	4	5
Been upset that my caree has changed so much from his or her former self?	1	2	3	4	5

If your score is under 20, you are doing okay. Between 20 and 45, you are experiencing some negative effects and need to remain vigilant. If you scored over 45, you might consider seeking help.

ASSESSING YOUR NEEDS

Can you or your caree…	Yes/No	Comments
Dress and undress without help?		
Drive or use public transportation on own?		
Shop for groceries or clothing on own?		
Prepare meals?		
Bathe or shower without help?		
Get in and out of bed without help?		
Be left alone during the day?		
Pay bills and manage finances on own?		
Clean the house?		
Manage household duties?		
Live alone comfortably and confidently?		
Remain active in life and hobbies?		
Walk, climb stairs and get around the house?		

DRIVING SKILLS ASSESSMENT

Did your loved one...	Yes or no?	Notes
Drive at inappropriate speeds?		
Ignore or misinterpret a traffic sign or light?		
Appear confused or scared?		
Stop in traffic for no reason?		
Have a near miss?		
Get lost on a familiar route?		
Have physical difficulty while driving (turning neck, etc.)?		
Mistake the gas and brake pedals for each other?		
Receive a traffic citation or warning?		

If your loved one has experienced any of these warning signs, it is time to have a difficult conversation. But, it could save their life and other innocent lives as well.

*The preceding checklists have been adapted from agis.com. For more checklists on hiring a home care agency, evaluating an assisted living facility, and much more, go to agis.com.

PREPARATION FOR INCAPACITATING AND END OF LIFE EVENTS

Proactive steps to consider for management of your health care, financial assets, and related legal issues.

Authorized Signer. Authorizes an individual to sign checks on your bank account(s), so he or she can pay bills and help manage your bank transactions. This person should be a trusted family member or friend, as this individual will be considered a co-owner and legally authorized to write checks and transfer money from your bank accounts.

Durable Power of Attorney. This legal instrument grants an individual power to manage your assets and other financial matters should you become incapacitated and to distribute assets after your death. Again, this should be a person you trust completely.

Health Care Directive. This a written document in which you appoint an individual to make health care decisions for you if you become unable to make them. These might include in-home care, assisted living facility or nursing home arrangements, and instructions for medical treatments by medical care professionals.

Advance Directive ("Living Will"). This document may also be included in your health care directive. It states your desire to die with dignity and directs physicians and other attending medical professionals to forego extraordinary, unnecessary life sustaining procedures.

Living Trust. This legal document allows you to transfer ownership and control of your assets to a trust, which can be irrevocable or revocable. A revocable living trust allows a designated "trustee" (usually you and or your spouse) to manage your assets during your lifetime and provides for how they will be distributed after you die. A revocable trust can be modified while you are alive but becomes irrevocable upon your death.

Author Page

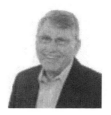

Jerry Gill retired from Oklahoma State University after serving thirty-four years in external relations positions, including twenty-two years as President and CEO of the OSU Alumni Association. He has a PhD in history and has taught history classes and authored academic articles and books.

Jerry resides west of Stillwater, Oklahoma, with his wife, Susan. They have four children and three grandchildren. He is active in the ministry of First United Methodist Church Stillwater and has taught an adult Sunday school class for nearly forty years.

Diagnosed with Parkinson's in 2010, Jerry is currently serving on the board of directors of the Parkinson Foundation of Oklahoma.

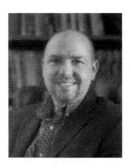

Bruce McIntyre currently serves as the Executive Director of the Parkinson Foundation of Oklahoma. As the author of *Graceful Transitions: An Inspirational Guide for Family Caregivers and Care Receivers*, Bruce shares his expert guidance and warm humor with thousands of people each year.

As a caregiver for his wife for the past 11 years, Bruce understands the world of chronic illness and caregiving. He has led the Caregiver Fundamentals Project in Oklahoma City and served caregivers as a business, church, and non-profit leader. Bruce is also the author of *Resilient Life* and he earned a Master of Divinity from Abilene Christian University. You can learn more about him at BruceMcIntyre.com or listen in on his Care Break podcast with Denise Brown at caregiving.com.

Made in the USA
San Bernardino, CA
27 July 2016